Fast Facts for the Primary FRCA and EDAIC

The Primary FRCA is a marathon exam that requires candidates to concentrate on solving MCQs first and then prepare for the OSCE and SOE viva. The EDAIC Part 1 involves MCQs, and Part 2 uses viva to test candidates. All these exams demand a strong knowledge of basic sciences relevant to anaesthesia. The *Fast Facts* content aids quick revision in the lead up to the examinations and maximises the chances of exam success.

Covering all the high-yield facts together with concept building, the content ensures that students benefit at all stages of their preparation, especially during the last few weeks before examinations. Past MCQs and core viva concepts have been presented in bullet points, tabular format and diagrams for easy assimilation. The Primary FRCA is shifting towards asking SBAs, and this book covers both the SBA and MTF formats of MCQs. It includes over 180 topics, and is subdivided into sections on Physiology, Pharmacology, Physics and Anatomy.

The key ingredient to get through any exam is confidence. By facilitating timely revision of the entire curriculum, this book makes sure that candidates for both the Primary FRCA and EDAIC will enter the examination hall with a positive mindset and comprehensive knowledge of the basic sciences required by anaesthetists.

Dr Amit Sharma is a specialty trainee in intensive care medicine and anaesthesia (dual CCT). He is currently working in Queen Elizabeth Hospital, Birmingham, UK. He did his graduation and post-graduation in anaesthesia from the prestigious Maulana Azad Medical College, New Delhi, which is one of the top three medical colleges in India. After that, he cleared EDAIC and registered with GMC to work as a Junior Specialist Doctor in the NHS. During this time, he completed his FRCA examination with distinction in both primary and final FRCA and joined training in the UK. He has an active interest in cardiac intensive care and well-being initiatives.

Fast Facts for the Primary FRCA and EDAIC

Basic Science for Anaesthetists

Amit Sharma

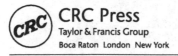

CRC Press
Taylor & Francis Group
Boca Raton London New York

CRC Press is an imprint of the
Taylor & Francis Group, an **informa** business

First edition published 2024
by CRC Press
6000 Broken Sound Parkway NW, Suite 300, Boca Raton, FL 33487-2742

and by CRC Press
4 Park Square, Milton Park, Abingdon, Oxon, OX14 4RN

CRC Press is an imprint of Taylor & Francis Group, LLC

© 2024 Amit Sharma

ISBN: 9781032486819 (hbk)
ISBN: 9781032483597 (pbk)
ISBN: 9781003390244 (ebk)

DOI: 10.1201/9781003390244

Typeset in Rotis Serif
by KnowledgeWorks Global Ltd.

Dedicated to:

My wife, Kritika Vats, who despite being tired of my numerous exams, still wanted me to write this book.

My daughter Aaryana Meera Sharma, who is more demanding than her mom, but has still cooperated equally for this book.

and

Above all, my parents, Mr. Viney Bhushan Sharma and Mrs. Sandhya Sharma for the infinite sacrifices they made for me.

Contents

Preface

Primary FRCA is a marathon exam that requires candidates to concentrate on solving MCQs first and then prepare for OSCE and SOE viva. EDAIC Part 1 involves MCQs and Part 2 uses viva to test candidates. All these exams demand a strong knowledge of basic sciences relevant to anaesthesia. During my preparation for these exams, I realized that the breadth of the course was huge and reading the textbooks towards the end was a daunting task. A book that would help candidates to revise quickly in the end was needed; hence, the idea to write this book was born.

The aim of this book is to amalgamate high-yield facts with concept building to make sure that students benefit at all stages of their preparation, especially during the last few weeks before examinations. Past MCQs and core viva concepts have been presented in bullet points, tabular form and diagrams to ensure that the book is helpful before both MCQs and viva. Primary FRCA is shifting towards asking SBAs, and this book covers both the SBA and MTF formats of MCQs.

Passing an examination mostly involves not getting the repeat questions wrong. By providing all the previously asked questions in bullet format instead of the cumbersome paragraph format, revision is done quickly and completely. This book is easily one of the most updated books on the market and will help candidates for many years to come.

The key ingredient to get through any exam is confidence before the exam. By facilitating timely revision of the entire curriculum, this book makes sure that you enter the examination hall with a positive mindset and then we all know what happens: "The whole universe conspires to get the job done for you."

Acknowledgements

First and foremost, I would like to thank all the endless examinations I had to go through for bringing out that nerdish streak in me; hence, I ended up writing a book.

A huge heartfelt thanks to my first educational supervisor and mentor in the UK, Dr Chetan Parcha, for his absolute support in helping me settle into the new NHS system. This made me dedicate my time to examinations with a happy mind and crack them without fear.

Every writer has an inspiration, and I would like to express my deepest gratitude to Dr Emma Plunkett, whose innate personality of being a wellbeing enthusiast was a motivation in writing this one. Like her, somebody who calmed nerves with her mere presence, I wanted to write a book to help slay some anxiety in those last few days before examinations.

I really appreciate the personalized efforts of Dr Tomasz Torlinski and Dr Randeep Mullhi in giving me the confidence to get through the grills of my initial days in intensive care.

A big shout out to all my fellow nurses, midwives and amazing ACCPs, junior doctors and consultants in the Department of Anaesthesia and Critical Care at Queen Elizabeth Hospital, Birmingham, for the never-ending love and affection that helped me complete this book. Special thanks to Dr Philip Moore, Dr Tessa Oelofse, Dr Tonny Veenith, Dr Ravi Hebbali, Dr Harjot Singh, Dr S Natarajan, Dr S Jagannathan, Dr Somasundaram Jeyanthan, Dr Ravi Chauhan, Dr Jeremy Marwick, Dr Laura Tasker, Dr Dhruv Parekh, Dr Shivanand Chavan, Dr David Balthazor, Dr Kerry Cullis, Dr Rajneesh Sachdeva, Dr Simon Smart, Dr Gauhar Sharih, Dr Yasmin Poonawala, Dr Jaimin Patel, Dr Mansoor Bangash, Dr Richard Browne, Dr Tiberiu Simu, Dr Annabelle Whapples, Dr John Kelly, Dr Asif Arshad, Dr Ciro Morgese, Dr Phillip El-Dalil, Dr Shraddha Goyal, Dr Julie Robin, Dr Phillip Howells, Dr Ranjna Basra, Dr Jignesh Patel, Dr Lyndon Harkett, Dr Melanie Sahni and Dr Claire Scanlon for taking very good care of me. Last but not the least, thanks to Dr Vinay Reddy-Kolanu for showing great interest in developing the physician in me.

Every building must have a foundation, and my working experience in India helped me prepare for the bigger challenges ahead. Special thanks to Dr Rakesh Kumar, Dr Panna Jain, Dr Kirti Nath Saxena, Dr Munisha Agarwal, Dr Anju Bhalotra, Dr Sonia Wadhawan, Dr Bharti Taneja, Dr Radha Gupta, Dr Abhijeet Khaund, Dr Monika Gupta, Dr Lalit Gupta, Dr Amit Kohli, Dr Saurabh Taneja, Dr Pooja Chopra Wadwa, Dr Munish Chauhan, Dr Manu Bhasin, Dr Sukhyanti Kerai and Dr Meghana Srivastava for always showing confidence in me.

All good acts have a strong supporting cast, and I would like to thank my father-in-law Mr Puneet Kumar Vats, my mother-in-law Udita Vats, my brother Ankit

Sharma, my sisters-in-law Kanika Vats and Noor Dharmarha, my brother-in-law Udbhav Vats and baby Saanvi for their unwavering support and assistance. This also makes sure that I avoid a civil war at home.

I will always be indebted to my best friend Supriya Chaudhary who would have been happy seeing me progress in life.

This acknowledgement can't be complete without the mention of my friends, Dr Sunny Yadav, Dr Swapnil Mahendrakar, Dr Pooja Sachdeva, Dr Romit Bhushan, Dr Mayank Chauhan, Dr Rahul Sapra, Dr Sadhana Saini, The G-gang, The Wilder animalzz, Dr Prameeta Jha, Dr Shalini Achra, Dr Abhishek Bansal, Dr Mrinal Yadava, Dr Anubha Khetarpaul, Dr Taru Jain, Dr Rohan Sikka and Dr Manan Bajaj for touching my life at various points of my journey and making it worthwhile.

Finally, the author would like to thank Miranda Bromage at Taylor & Francis/CRC Press for her constant positive words that helped to make this book a reality. She always gave me that extra assurance that a first-time writer needs. Hopefully we get to collaborate more in future.

PHYSIOLOGY

Respiratory System

Tracheobronchial tree

- **Trachea:** C6 to T4, 10–12 cm length, ciliated columnar epithelium
- **Bronchi:** Right main bronchus 25° from trachea, left main bronchus 45° from trachea
- **Small bronchi:** Cuboidal epithelium
- **Terminal bronchioles:** Diameter <1 mm. Devoid of the alveoli and cartilage. **Abundant smooth muscle**
- **Respiratory bronchioles:** *Intermittent alveoli. Gas exchange starts*
- **Alveolar ducts:** Continuous alveoli
- 300 million alveoli, 50–100 m² surface area. ***Type II alveolar cells produce surfactant***
- **Bronchopulmonary segments:** Right side (10)
  - **Right upper lobe:** Apical, anterior, posterior
  - **Right middle lobe:** Medial, lateral
  - **Right lower lobe:** Apical, anterior basal, posterior basal, medial basal, lateral basal
- **Bronchopulmonary segments:** Left side (10)
  - **Left upper lobe:** Apical, anterior, posterior
  - **Left lingular lobe:** Superior, inferior
  - **Left lower lobe:** Apical, anterior basal, posterior basal, medial basal, lateral basal

Right upper lobe bronchus branches at 90° posteriorly to the main right bronchus. Hence, foreign body or fluid aspirated by a patient in supine position enters the right upper lobe.

Lung volumes and capacities

- **Lung volumes:** Measured using spirometer
- **Lung capacity:** Sum of two or more volumes
- **Tidal volume (TV):** Volume of air inspired during a normal breath. 500 mL

DOI: 10.1201/9781003390244-2

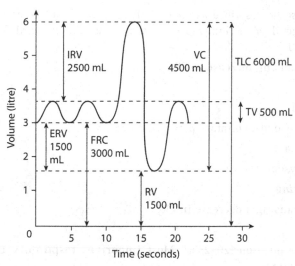

Figure 1.1   Spirometry.

- **Inspiratory reserve volume (IRV):** Volume of air that can be inspired above the normal TV. 2500 mL
- **Expiratory reserve volume (ERV):** Volume of air that can be expired after the normal TV. 1500 mL
- **Residual volume (RV):** Volume of air that remains in lungs after breathing out ERV. 1500 mL
- **Functional residual capacity (FRC):** Volume of air remaining in the lung after a normal TV breath. FRC = ERV + RV. 3000 mL
- **Inspiratory capacity (IC):** Maximum volume of air that can be inspired after expiration of a normal TV breath. IC = TV + IRV. 3000 mL
- **Expiratory capacity (EC):** Maximum volume of air that can be expired after inspiration of a normal TV breath. EC = TV + ERV. 3000 mL
- **Vital capacity (VC):** Maximal volume that can be expired after a maximal inspiration. VC = ERV + TV + IRV. 4500 mL
- **Total lung capacity (TLC):** Volume of air in lungs after maximal inspiration. TLC = RV + VC. 6000 mL
- TV, IRV and ERV can be measured using a spirometer. *RV and FRC can be measured using body plethysmography and helium dilution technique*

Functional residual capacity

- FRC is defined as the volume of air remaining in the lung after a normal TV breath. FRC = ERV + RV = 3000 mL

- It can also be described as volume of air in the lungs when the inward elastic recoil of the lungs is exactly same as the outward force of the chest wall
- **Factors causing increase in FRC**
  - Males
  - Height
  - Positive end-expiratory pressure (PEEP)
  - Asthma
  - Emphysema
  - *Standing*
- **Factors causing a decrease in FRC**
  - Age
  - Supine position (20–25%). **Most important respiratory change on lying down**
  - Pregnancy (20–30% at term)
  - Obesity
  - Anaesthesia
- **Closing capacity:** Volume of lungs at which the *smaller airway collapses* during expiration. In a *supine person aged 44 years and a standing person aged 66 years, closing capacity is equal to FRC*

  Once the closing capacity is more than FRC, gas trapping happens.
  - *Closing capacity = Residual volume + Closing volume*

Flow volume loops

- Spirometry is used to create flow volume loops
  - Expiratory flow is above X-axis
  - Inspiratory flow is below X-axis
- **Mechanism**
  - Patient takes a VC breath before starting the test, thus reaching TLC
  - Patient then takes a forced expiration, and a loop is drawn clockwise from TLC
  - Loop rises rapidly to a flow rate of 8–10 L/s
  - The inspiratory limb is square-shaped and maximum flow of 4–6 L/s. The direction of the loop is anticlockwise and moves from RV to TLC
- **Obstructive disease:** e.g., *COPD/asthma*. Peak expiratory flow rate (PEFR) is decreased, and RV is increased by gas trapping

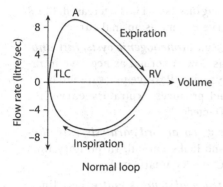

Normal loop

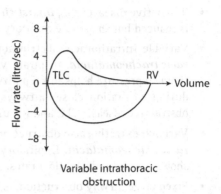

Variable intrathoracic obstruction

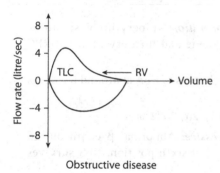

Obstructive disease

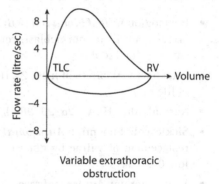

Variable extrathoracic obstruction

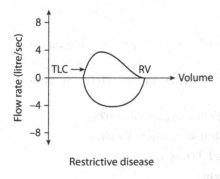

Restrictive disease

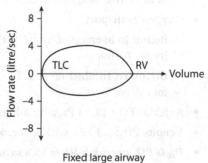

Fixed large airway obstruction

Figure 1.2   Flow volume loops.

- Restrictive disease: e.g., *interstitial lung disease*. TLC is decreased. PEFR is reduced but shape of expiratory curve is same as normal curve
- Variable intrathoracic obstruction: e.g., *bronchogenic cysts, intrathoracic tracheomalacia.* Inspiratory gas flow is normal as negative intrathoracic pressure helps to keep airways open. Positive pressure produced during expiration closes airways and produces expiratory curve-like obstructive disease. TLC and RV unaffected
- Variable extrathoracic obstruction: e.g., *vocal cord paralysis, extrathoracic tracheomalacia*. Expiratory limb looks normal. Inspiratory limb shows marked reduced flow rates. TLC and RV unaffected
- Fixed large airway obstruction: e.g., *tracheal stenosis, goitre.* Both limbs have reduced flow. TLC and RV unaffected

Oxyhaemoglobin dissociation curve (OHDC)

- Haemoglobin: *Red blood cell (RBC) formation* – proerythroblast, prorubricyte, rubricyte, normoblast, reticulocyte and then erythroblast. RBC survives for 120 days
- Fetal haemoglobin (HbF): 2α, 2γ. HbF changes to HbA at around 6 months of life
- Normal adult HbA_1: *2α, 2β (98%), HbA_2: 2α, 2δ* (2%)
- Sickle cell anaemia: *Autosomal recessive:* Abnormal β chain due to replacement of valine by glutamic acid at sixth position. HbS survives for 10–20 days
- Thalassaemia: *Autosomal recessive:* reduced rate of synthesis of one of the globin chains
- Methaemoglobinemia: Normal oxygen binds to Fe^{2+} but no oxidation happens, and iron remains in Fe^{2+} (ferrous form). Fe^{2+} is oxidised into Fe^{3+} form in methaemoglobinemia
- Oxygen transport
  - Bound to haemoglobin: 97%. Haemoglobin $\uparrow$ oxygen-carrying capacity by 70-fold
  - Dissolved in plasma: 3%. This fraction triggers the hypoxic respiratory drive
- Arterial PO_2: 13.3 kPa with a haemoglobin saturation of 97%
- Venous PO_2: 5.3 kPa with a haemoglobin saturation of 75%
- *P_{50} is PO_2 at which Hb is 50% saturated.* PO_2 is 3.5 kPa
- Factors that shift the OHDC to the right
  - Acidosis

- o Hyperthermia
- o ↑2,3-diphosphoglyceric acid (DPG)
- o Hypercapnia
- o *Anaemia*
- o HbS
- o Pregnancy
- Factors that shift the OHDC to the left
  - o Alkalosis
  - o Hypothermia
  - o ↓2,3 DPG
  - o Hypocapnia
  - o Methaemoglobin
  - o Carboxyhaemoglobin (Hb + CO, 200 times more affinity to Hb than O_2)
  - o HbF
- Shape of OHDC: Sigmoid
  - o **Allosteric modulation:** As O_2 binds to haemoglobin, haem moieties assume a 'relaxed' or R state. When oxygen dissociates, the reverse happens, and haem moieties take up a 'tense' or T state
  - o **Cooperative binding:** O_2 binding to haemoglobin leads to increased affinity of haemoglobin for additional O_2 molecules
- Myoglobin dissociation curve (MDC)
  - o Single polypeptide with a haem ring found in skeletal muscle
  - o Higher affinity for O_2 than haemoglobin, hence, rectangular parabola shape

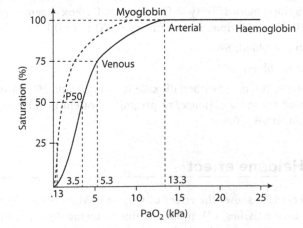

Figure 1.3   OHDC and MDC.

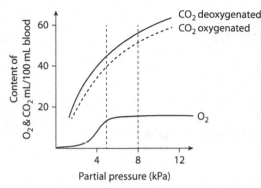

Figure 1.4 CO_2 dissociation curve.

Carbon dioxide dissociation curve

- Carbon dioxide transport
  - Dissolved CO_2 in plasma: Carbon dioxide is 20 times more soluble than oxygen in plasma
    - Arterial blood: 5%
    - Venous blood: 10%
  - Carbonic acid: Carbon dioxide combines with water to form carbonic acid, a reaction catalysed by carbonic anhydrase. **Most important mechanisms for transport**
    - Arterial blood: 90%
    - Venous blood: 60%
  - Haemoglobin bound: Carbaminohaemoglobin (Hb + CO_2). Haemoglobin has 3.5 times more affinity to CO_2 than O_2. Carboxyhaemoglobin is Hb + CO (Hb has 200 times more affinity to CO than O_2)
    - Arterial blood: 5%
    - Venous blood: 30%
- Every minute, 200 mL of carbon dioxide is exhaled, and 250 mL of oxygen is consumed per minute. Hence, respiratory quotient (RQ) is CO_2 production/O_2 consumed = 0.8

Bohr and Haldane effect

- **Bohr effect:** This shows the effect of CO_2 on oxygen transport. In metabolically active tissues, CO_2 produced due to metabolism combines with water to form carbonic acid. Carbonic acid dissociates into hydrogen ions and bicarbonate. Hydrogen ions decrease blood pH. This acidotic environment favours reduced affinity of oxygen to haemoglobin. This causes unloading of oxygen

$$CO_2 + H_2O \rightarrow H_2CO_3 \rightarrow H^+ + HCO_3^- \rightarrow H^+ + HbO_2 \rightarrow HHb + O_2$$

- **Double Bohr effect:** In placenta, oxygen and carbon dioxide are exchanged due to the Bohr effect. The fetal side releases CO_2 towards the maternal side. This CO_2 results in the release of oxygen from maternal haemoglobin (Bohr effect). The decrease in CO_2 on the fetal side leads to oxygen loading
- **Haldane effect:** This shows the effect of O_2 on carbon dioxide transport. As blood enters the pulmonary circulation, O_2 diffuses across the RBC membrane and binds to haemoglobin. The binding of O_2 leads to allosteric changes in haemoglobin (T state to the R state) with loss of H^+ and CO_2
- **Hamburger effect/chloride shift:** This involves the exchange of bicarbonate and chloride ions across the membrane of RBCs. The carbon dioxide is taken up by the RBCs, and the carbonic anhydrase enzyme converts CO_2 into H_2CO_3. This H_2CO_3 divides into H^+ and HCO_3^- Chloride anions (Cl^-) from plasma enter cytoplasm of RBCs along with diffusion of bicarbonate ($HCO3^-$) out of cytoplasm of erythrocytes (RBCs) into the blood plasma. Most of the free hydrogen cations react with reduced haemoglobin. This serves to maintain the electrochemical neutrality in RBCs or maintaining the blood pH

Control of ventilation

- Ventilation is controlled by three main components:
  - *Control centre: Brainstem*
    - **Dorsal respiratory group (DRG) of neurons:** Medulla and controls inspiration
    - **Ventral respiratory group (VRG) of neurons:** Medulla and controls expiration
    - **Pneumotaxic area:** Located in the pons. Assists in fine-tuning inspiration. Inspiration can be prematurely terminated by the pneumotaxic centre
  - *Effectors: Respiratory muscles*
    - Inspiration is active and facilitated by the diaphragm ($C_{3,4,5}$), intercostals, abdominal muscles and accessory muscles
    - Expiration is mostly passive

- ○ *Sensors: Chemoreceptors*
  - ♦ **Central chemoreceptors:** Ventral surface of the medulla. Responds mostly to H^+ ions and is the most important factor that changes minute ventilation. Cerebrospinal fluid (CSF) has less buffering capacity than the blood; hence, H^+ ions act faster
  - ♦ **Peripheral chemoreceptors:** Carotid bodies at bifurcation of the common carotid artery (via **glossopharyngeal nerve**). Aortic bodies along the arch of the aorta (via **vagus** nerve). Responds to O_2 tension mainly, and CO_2 and H^+ are weak stimulants
    - – **Blood supply to carotid bodies is 2000 mL/100 g/min**
  - ♦ **Chemical and irritant receptors:** In mucosa of upper airway, they initiate laryngeal closure as a reflex to inhalation of injurious substances. Hyperventilation in response to noxious gases
  - ♦ **Pressure receptors:** In smooth muscles, they help to control the depth of respiration
  - ♦ **Lung stretch receptors/*Hering–Breuer reflex:*** In smooth muscles, they inhibit inspiration in response to distension of lung by increasing expiratory rate
  - ♦ **J or juxtacapillary receptors:** Found in alveoli, responds to fluid in capillaries (pulmonary oedema) by causing tachypnoea
  - ♦ **Joint and muscle receptors:** Influence ventilation in response to exercise

Hypoxia

- **Hypoxia:** Insufficient oxygen supply or inability to utilize oxygen at cellular level. Can be divided into four groups
- **Hypoxic hypoxia:** *Reduction in partial pressure of oxygen in blood. Causes include:*
  - ○ Low FiO_2
  - ○ **Hypoventilation:** Central nervous system (CNS) depression, disorders of the respiratory muscles
  - ○ **Diffusion impairment:** Pulmonary oedema, pneumonia
  - ○ **Ventilation-perfusion mismatch:** chronic obstructive pulmonary disease (COPD), asthma
- **Anaemic hypoxia:** Inadequate oxygen-carrying capacity of blood
  - ○ Low haemoglobin levels
  - ○ *Carbon monoxide poisoning*
- **Stagnant hypoxia:** Inadequate tissue oxygenation due to failure of perfusion
  - ○ Cardiogenic shock

- **Histotoxic hypoxia:** Inability of the tissues to utilize the oxygen at a cellular mitochondrial level. Normal PaO_2
  - Cyanide poisoning

	PaO$_2$ (arterial oxygen)	PvO$_2$ (venous oxygen)
Normal	13.3 kPa	5.3 kPa
Hypoxic hypoxia	↓	↓
Anaemic hypoxia	Normal	↓
Stagnant hypoxia	Normal	↓
Histotoxic hypoxia	Normal	↑

$$\text{Oxygen Content} = [\text{Bound Oxygen}] + [\text{Dissolved Oxygen}]$$
$$= [Hb + 1.34 \times SpO_2] + [PaO_2 \times 0.0225]$$

- Arterial hypoxaemia causes vasoconstriction, whereas hypercapnia causes vasodilation
- **Carbon monoxide poisoning will cause lactic acidosis**

Ventilation and perfusion

- **Blood flow in lungs**
  - In the standing person, the blood flow decreases linearly from the bottom to the top
  - In the lying-down person, the posterior part of the lungs will have more blood flow than the anterior region
- **Ventilation in lungs**
  - The bases of the lung VENTILATE better than the upper zones. **The apices of lung are more expanded**
  - At the apex of the lungs, intrapleural pressure is –10 cm H_2O. Therefore, at rest, the apex of lungs has a large volume of air in alveoli
  - At the base of the lungs, intrapleural pressure is –2.5 cm H_2O. Therefore, at rest, the base of lungs has a low volume of air to start with. During inspiration, a large change of volume happens, and ventilation is better than apex
  - **Pleural pressure is between –3 and –5 cm H_2O**
- **Ventilation/Perfusion:** Differences in blood flow from the top of the lungs to the bottom vary more compared with changes in ventilation, hence, an upward sloping sigmoid curve

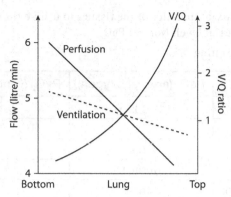

Figure 1.5   V/Q curve.

- **West zones:** The lung can be divided into three regions according to the dynamics between alveolar pressure (P_A), arterial pressure (P_a) and venous pressure (P_v)
  - **Zone 1:** (Dead-space ventilation). Apex of the lung. $P_A > P_a > P_v$. V/Q ratio is 3
  - **Zone 2:** Optimal ventilation-perfusion matching. $P_a > P_A > P_v$. V/Q ratio is 0.8
  - **Zone 3:** (Shunt). Base of the lung. $P_a > P_v > P_A$. V/Q ratio is 0.3
- **Dead-space ventilation:** Volume of air during inspiration that does not take part in gas exchange. *Physiological dead space = Anatomical dead space + Alveolar dead space*
  - **Anatomical dead space:** Volume of air in the conducting airways. 150 mL
  - **Alveolar dead space:** Part of alveoli which is ventilated but not perfused
- **Anatomical dead space:** *Fowler's method.* **Closing volume can also be measured**
  - 100% oxygen is maximally inspired at the end of a normal expiration
  - Slow exhalation is done through a nitrogen analyser, and nitrogen concentration is plotted against time
  - **In phase 1:** No nitrogen is expired initially, as conducting airways only has oxygen
  - **In phase 2:** Air from alveoli starts coming, and nitrogen concentration slowly increases
  - **In phase 3:** This is a plateau phase, where the alveolar gas containing nitrogen is exhaled
  - The curve is sigmoid in shape, and anatomical dead space can be calculated by drawing a vertical line through the curve

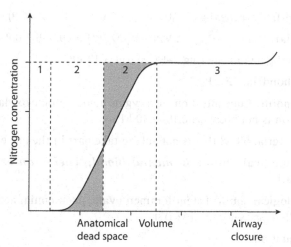

Figure 1.6   Anatomical dead space.

- Physiological dead space: *Bohr method*
  - The principle is that expired carbon dioxide is only from alveolar gas and not from the dead space. Hence, expired carbon dioxide is the sum of inspired carbon dioxide plus alveolar carbon dioxide
  - $V_D/V_T = P_ACO_2 - P_ECO_2/P_ACO_2$

    where V_D is dead-space volume, V_T is tidal volume, P_ACO_2 is alveolar carbon dioxide and P_ECO_2 is expired carbon dioxide
  - Physiological dead space ↑ with general anaesthesia

Alveolar gas equation and shunt

- **Alveolar gas equation:** This tells the partial pressure gradient driving oxygen across the alveolar-capillary membrane
  - $P_AO_2 = F_iO_2 (P_{ATM} - SVP) - P_ACO_2/RQ$

    where P_AO_2 is alveolar partial pressure of oxygen, F_iO_2 is the fraction of inspired oxygen, P_{ATM} is atmospheric pressure, SVP is saturated vapour pressure, P_ACO_2 is alveolar partial pressure of carbon dioxide and RQ is respiratory quotient
- **RQ:** Amount of carbon dioxide produced divided by oxygen consumed

$$RQ = CO_2/O_2$$

- **Oxygen cascade:** Stepwise reduction in oxygen partial pressure starting at inspired gas until the oxygen reaches the tissues
  - **Dry atmospheric gas:** $P_{ATM} \times F_iO_2 = 101.32 \times 20.93\% = 21.2$ kPa

- ○ Humidified tracheal gas: $F_iO_2 (P_{ATM} - SVP) = (101.32-6.3) = 19.9$ kPa
- ○ Alveolar gas: $F_iO_2 (P_{ATM} - SVP) - P_ACO_2/RQ = 19.9-5.3/0.8 = 13.3$ kPa
- ○ Arterial gas: Considering 2–5% shunt = 13 kPa
- ○ Mitochondria: 1.5 kPa
- **Pasteur point:** Concentration of oxygen below which oxidative phosphorylation is not possible. 0.15–0.30 kPa
- **Shunt:** Arterial blood that is not able to take part in the gas exchange
  - ○ **Physiological shunt:** *Bronchial blood, Thebesian veins.* 2–5% normally
  - ○ **Pathological shunt:** Patent foramen ovale, pneumonia, acute respiratory distress syndrome (ARDS)
- Shunt equation
  - ○ $Q_S/Q_T = (C_cO_2 - C_aO_2)/(C_cO_2 - C_vO_2)$

    where Q_S is shunted blood, Q_T is cardiac output, C_cO_2 is capillary oxygen concentration, C_aO_2 is arterial oxygen concentration and C_vO_2 is mixed venous oxygen concentration

Equations used in respiratory physiology

- Oxygen Content = [Bound Oxygen] + [Dissolved Oxygen]

    $$= [Hb + 1.34 \times SpO_2] + [PaO_2 \times 0.0225]$$
- Henderson–Hasselbach equation: pH = pKa + Log [conjugate base/acid]

    $$= pKa + Log [A^-]/[HA]$$
- **Bohr method:** Dead-space volume
  - ○ $V_D/V_T = P_ACO_2 - P_ECO_2/P_ACO_2$

    where V_D is dead-space volume, V_T is tidal volume, P_ACO_2 is alveolar carbon dioxide, P_ECO_2 is expired carbon dioxide
- **Alveolar gas equation:** This tells the partial pressure gradient driving oxygen across the alveolar-capillary membrane
  - ○ $P_AO_2 = F_iO_2 (P_{ATM} - SVP) - P_ACO_2/RQ$

    where P_AO_2 is alveolar partial pressure of oxygen,

    F_iO_2 is fraction of inspired oxygen,

    P_{ATM} is atmospheric pressure,

    SVP is saturated vapour pressure,

P_ACO_2 is alveolar partial pressure of carbon dioxide,

RQ is respiratory quotient.

- Shunt equation
  - $Q_S/Q_T = (C_cO_2 - C_aO_2)/(C_cO_2 - C_vO_2)$

  where Q_S is shunted blood,

  Q_T is cardiac output,

  C_cO_2 is capillary oxygen concentration,

  C_aO_2 is arterial oxygen concentration,

  C_vO_2 is mixed venous oxygen concentration.

One-lung ventilation

- Hypoxic pulmonary vasoconstriction (HPV): Protective reflex that diverts blood flow away from collapsed areas of lungs to better-ventilated ones
  - This starts within seconds of decrease in pO_2 of alveolar gas, and within minutes lobar blood flow is halved
  - Biphasic response with peaks at 5–20 min and 60–120 min due to increase in the intracellular calcium
  - Fall in alveolar PO_2 leads to less nitric oxide (NO) being synthesised and, hence, vasoconstriction
  - HPV increased by acidosis and hypercarbia, and decreased by alkalosis, hypocarbia, bronchodilators, vasodilators and volatile anaesthetic agents
  - **Pulmonary vascular resistance (PVR) is lowest at FRC and is high at both high and low lung volumes**
  - **HPV decreases physiological dead space**
- One-lung ventilation (OLV): Depends upon lateral decubitus position, open chest and collapse of non-dependent lung, all of which cause increased shunt
  - During two-lung ventilation in the lateral position, blood flow to the non-dependent lung is 40% compared with 60% to the dependent lung
  - 5% physiological shunt in lateral position in each lung makes it effectively 35% blood flow in non-dependent lung compared with 55% in dependent lung

- OLV creates at least a 50% shunt, hence, blood flow to the non-dependent lung becomes halved, 35/2 = 17.5%. As this blood goes to dependent lung, it now has 55 + 17.5 = 72.5% blood flow
- Therefore, the dependent lung gets 72.5% of the blood flow, but compliance is decreased because of the elevated diaphragm, and pressure from abdominal and mediastinal structures. This causes a V/Q mismatch
- **Hypoxemia during OLA**
  - Increase FiO_2 to 1.0
  - Check double-lumen tube (DLT) for cuff hernia/block/kink
  - Check anaesthetic circuit and connections
  - Check DLT position with fibreoptic scope
  - Ensure adequate cardiac output
  - Insufflate O_2 to non-ventilated lung
  - **Apply continuous positive airway pressure (CPAP) to non-ventilated lung: 5–10 cm H_2O**
  - Apply PEEP to ventilated lung
  - Intermittent insufflation of non-ventilated lung
  - Clamping appropriate pulmonary artery to reduce shunt

Respiratory compliance and resistance

- **Compliance:** Change in volume of lungs for a unit change in pressure
  - Respiratory compliance can be divided into lung compliance and thoracic wall compliance
  - 1/Respiratory compliance = 1/Lung compliance + 1/Thoracic wall compliance
  - Lung compliance = 200 mL/cm H_2O. Thoracic wall compliance = 200 mL/cm H_2O
  - *Respiratory compliance = 100 mL/cm H_2O*
  - **Static compliance:** Change in volume of lungs for a unit change in pressure when there is no airflow
  - **Dynamic compliance:** Change in volume of lungs for a unit change in pressure is plotted continuously throughout the respiratory cycle
  - The dynamic compliance is always lower than static compliance
  - Compliance ↓ in pulmonary oedema and fibrosis
  - *Compliance ↑ in emphysema and **elderly***

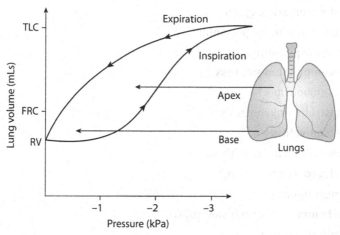

Figure 1.7   Lung pressure-volume loop.

- Resistance
  - Total resistance = airway resistance (80%) + tissue resistance (20%)
  - Airway resistance can be calculated using a **body plethysmograph**
  - As lungs collapse and volume reduces, airway resistance increases
  - **Airway resistance is increased in forced expiration and turbulence airflow**
- **Surface tension:** Force in dynes acting on an imaginary line 1.0 cm long within the liquid surface
  - Laplace's law, $P = 4 \times Ts/r$; where Ts is surface tension and r is radius
  - The liquid-lined alveoli have only 1 liquid/air interface, therefore, $P = 2 \, Ts/r$
- **Surfactant:** This lowers the surface tension. Surfactants increase compliance and prevent collapsing of alveoli
  - Composed of dipalmitoyl phosphatidyl choline (DPPC), a phospholipid
  - Synthesised in type II alveolar cells, granular pneumocytes
  - The elimination half-life, $t_{1/2} \sim 14$ hours

Hyperbaric oxygen

- **Hyperbaric oxygen:** Oxygen at greater than atmospheric pressure, usually 2–3 atmospheres
- Dissolved oxygen
  - 21% O_2 at 1 atmosphere in 100 mL blood = 0.3 mL O_2
  - 100% O_2 at 3 atmospheres in 100 mL blood = 5.7 mL

- Use of hyperbaric oxygen
  - Carbon monoxide poisoning
  - Cyanide poisoning
  - **Decompression sickness**
  - Air embolism
  - Clostridial myonecrosis
  - **Osteomyelitis**
  - Jehovah's witness with anaemia
  - Delayed wound healing
  - Crush injury
  - **Ischemia and reperfusion injury**
  - Radiation injury
  - Thermal burns
- Side effects of hyperbaric oxygen
  - Lung damage
  - Sinus and middle ear damage
  - Changes in vision, causing nearsightedness or myopia
  - Seizures

Altitude

- **High altitude:** >2500 m above sea level, extreme altitude >6000 m, Mount Everest is 8848 m high
- **Body compensatory changes**
  - **Hyperventilation:** Fall in PaO_2 below 8 kPa, stimulates the peripheral chemoreceptors. **Acute response to altitude**
  - **Sinus tachycardia:** Sympathetic stimulation
  - **HPV:** It optimizes V/Q matching
  - **Leftward shift of the OHDC:** 2,3 DPG production increases
  - **Polycythaemia:** Increased erythropoietin secretion
  - **Hypercoagulability:** Due to increased haematocrit
- **Acute high-altitude illness**
  - **Acute mountain sickness (AMS):** Neurological constellation of symptoms
    - Nausea, headache, fatigue, dizziness, sleep disturbance
    - Symptoms improve after 3–4 days at the same altitude

o High–altitude cerebral oedema (HACE): Severe form of AMS, can lead to coma

   ◆ Due to vasodilation of cerebral vessels in response to hypoxia

o High–altitude pulmonary oedema (HAPE): Due to severe HPV

   ◆ Persistent dry cough, fever, severe dyspnoea at rest

o Treatment: Descent, oxygen, hyperbaric chamber, acetazolamide, nifedipine and dexamethasone

- Effect on anaesthetic equipment at high altitude

o Variable bypass vaporiser: *Partial pressure of the volatile agent remains the same*

   ◆ SVP of the volatile agent remains the same

   ◆ Therefore, same settings as at sea level

o Measured flow vaporiser (desflurane): Partial pressure is halved as measured flow

   ◆ Concentration on dial should be increased compared with concentration at sea levels

o Flowmeters: Gases have a lower density

   ◆ Underread at high altitude

o Bourdon pressure gauge: Overreads at higher altitude

o Venturi-type O_2 masks: Deliver higher percentage of O_2 than at sea level

o Gas and vapour analysers: Underread

Diving

- Diving: Barometric pressure increases by 1 atmosphere for every 10 m descent

- Diving reflex: Cardiopulmonary changes

o Apnoea: To prevent the lungs from filling with water

o Bradycardia: Due to vagus nerve

o Peripheral vasoconstriction: Blood diverted from peripheries to maximise heart perfusion

- Breath-hold diving

o Increased density of inhaled gas: Turbulent gas flow leading to increased work of breathing

o Nitrogen narcosis: High pressures of N_2 can directly cause CNS symptoms like euphoria, incoordination, coma

- o **Oxygen toxicity:** O_2 at high pressures can cause acute lung injury, seizures and loss of consciousness
- **Decompression sickness:** *At* depths above 20 m, nitrogen is absorbed into tissues
  - o Problems occur during rapid ascent
  - o Pneumothorax or perforated tympanic membrane
  - o **Joint pain:** Called 'the bends'
  - o **Pulmonary circulation:** Dyspnoea (the chokes) and retrosternal pain
  - o **Arterial circulation:** Gas embolism
  - o Using a non-air gas mixture such as helium/oxygen mixture reduces the risk of decompression sickness
- **Drowning:** Primary respiratory impairment due to submersion in a liquid medium
  - o Classification of drowning
    - ◆ **Class 1:** No evidence of aspiration
    - ◆ **Class 2:** Evidence of aspiration but with adequate ventilation
    - ◆ **Class 3:** Evidence of aspiration with inadequate ventilation
    - ◆ **Class 4:** Absent ventilation and circulation
  - o **CVS effects:** Diving reflex with massive catecholamine surge causing arrhythmias, pulmonary oedema
  - o **CNS effects:** Hypoxic brain injury starts within 5 min
  - o **Metabolic effects:** Hypothermia
  - o **Infections:** *Staphylococcus aureus, Pseudomonas, Aspergillus*

Cardiovascular System

2

Coronary circulation

- Coronary circulation: 5% of the cardiac output = 250 mL/min
  - At rest, heart extracts 70% of the oxygen content of the arterial blood
  - Blood flows mostly during diastole
- Right coronary artery: Arises from anterior aortic sinus supplies
  - Sinoatrial (SA) node in 60% of people
  - Atrioventricular (AV) node in 90% of people
  - Right atrium
  - Right ventricle
  - Diaphragmatic surface of the left ventricle
  - Posterior one-third of the septum
- Left coronary artery: Arises from left posterior aortic sinus supplies
  - SA node in 40% of people
  - Left atrium
  - Left ventricle
  - Anterior two-thirds of the septum
- Venous system: *Two main routes* – Greater cardiac and smaller cardiac venous system
  - Greater cardiac venous system: 75% of the deoxygenated blood
    - *Coronary sinus:* Largest cardiac vein. Drains into right atrium. Formed by tributaries like great cardiac vein and left marginal vein, both of which follow the course of left coronary artery. Other tributaries are middle cardiac vein, small cardiac vein and right marginal vein which follows the course of right coronary artery
    - *Anterior cardiac veins:* Flows directly into right atrium
  - Smaller cardiac venous system: 25% of deoxygenated blood
    - *Thebesian veins:* Flows directly into all heart chambers. **True, anatomical shunt.** Minimal proportion
- Nervous system: Superficial and deep cardiac plexus
  - Sympathetic nervous system: *Preganglionic:* T1–T5
    - Postganglionic: Cervical sympathetic
  - Parasympathetic nervous system: Vagus nerve

DOI: 10.1201/9781003390244-3

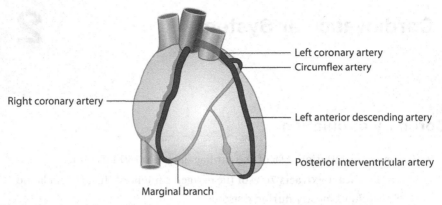

Figure 2.1 Arterial system.

- **Regulation of coronary blood flow**
  - ○ **Intrinsic control**
    1. **Metabolic:** H^+, K^+, adenosine and CO_2 cause vasodilation
    2. **Myogenic**
    3. **Endothelial:** Nitric oxide (NO) and prostacyclin (PGI_2) causes vasodilation. Thromboxane A_2 produces vasoconstriction
  - ○ **Extrinsic control**
    1. **Neurogenic: Autonomic nervous system:** Sympathetic nervous system and parasympathetic nervous system
    2. **Humoral control:** Vasodilators like atrial natriuretic peptide and vasoconstrictors like vasopressin and angiotensin II
- **Adrenaline is used in Advanced Life Support (ALS) because it increases perfusion of the coronary arteries and brain**

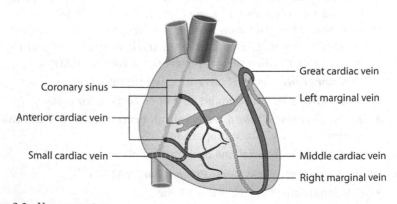

Figure 2.2 Venous system.

Electrocardiogram and cardiac axis

- Electrocardiogram (ECG): Test used to measure the electrical activity of a person's heart
  - Normal axis: –30° to +90°
    - *Normal axis:* Positive QRS in leads I, II and III
    - *Right axis deviation:* Between +90° and +180°. Negative QRS in lead I
    - *Left axis deviation:* Between –30° and –90°. Negative QRS in lead III
  - Speed of paper: 25 mm/s, 10 mm = 1 mV, one large square = 5 mm
  - Ischemia detection: *Lead II:* 35%, *V5:* 75%, *II + V5:* 90%
- Morphology and intervals
  - P wave: Atrial depolarisation
  - PR interval: Start of P wave to end of the PR segment. Normal value 0.12–0.2 s
  - QRS wave: Ventricular depolarisation. Normal value is <0.12 s
  - T wave: Ventricular repolarisation
  - ST segment: Junction of QRS complex and ST segment to beginning of T wave. Isoelectric normally
  - QT interval: Start of QRS complex to end of T wave. QTc is prolonged if >440 ms in men or >460 ms in women
- Components of ECG machine
  - A detection device
    - Electrodes are detection devices. Made up of silver/silver chloride
    - Resistance in each lead of ECG reducing current flow and risk of a harmful current
  - A transducer
  - An amplifier
  - A display device
- Patterns in ECG
  - S1Q3T3: Pulmonary embolism
  - U wave: Hypokalaemia
  - *Tall T waves: Hyperkalaemia – Give calcium gluconate immediately*
  - J wave or Osborn wave: Hypothermia
  - Delta wave: Wolff–Parkinson–White syndrome
  - Trifascicular block: Right bundle branch block (RBBB) + left anterior hemiblock (LAHB) + ↑PR interval
  - Left ventricular (LV) hypertrophy: S wave in V1 + R wave in V6 > 35 mm

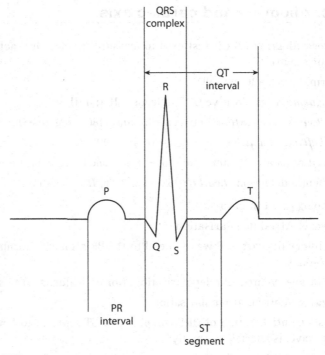

Figure 2.3   ECG.

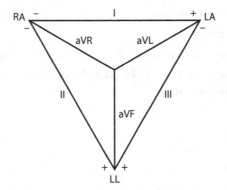

Figure 2.4   Einthoven's triangle.

Cardiac cycle

- The cardiac cycle can be divided into systole and diastole
- **Systole has two stages:** Isovolumetric contraction and ejection
- **Diastole has four stages:** Isovolumetric relaxation, rapid ventricular filling, slow ventricular filling, atrial contraction

- Stages
  - Atrial contraction: During late diastole, atrium contracts and contributes to 30% of ventricular filling. 'a' wave in central venous pressure (CVP) is produced due to back pressure in veins
  - Isovolumetric contraction: This is the start of systole. All valves are closed. Pressure in ventricle rises from baseline. The first heart sound is heard due to closing of mitral and tricuspid valve. 'c' wave in CVP is produced due to bulging of tricuspid valve
    - A decrease in preload decreases LV fibre length and hence LV end-diastolic volume (Frank–Starling law)
  - Ejection: As the ventricle pressure exceeds the pressure in aorta and pulmonary artery (PA), ejection of blood happens as aortic and pulmonic valve open. Around 65–70 mL of blood is ejected; this is known as the stroke volume (SV), with 60 mL blood remaining in the ventricle
  - Isovolumetric relaxation: Both the aortic and pulmonic valve close producing second heart sound. Now both the ventricles relax with all valves closed
  - Rapid ventricular filling: Mitral and tricuspid valves open causing rapid movement of blood in ventricles due to suction forces produced by opening of valves
  - Slow ventricular filling: Rapid phase is followed by slow passive filling of ventricle during diastole
- Ejection fraction is one of the best measures of LV contractility
- **The base of epicardium is the last part of ventricle to be depolarised**

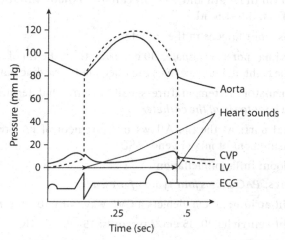

Figure 2.5   Cardiac cycle.

CVP waveform vs pulmonary artery catheter (PAC) waveform

- **CVP waveform:** Pressure recorded from the right atrium or superior vena cava and is representative of the filling pressure of the right side of the heart
  - Normal is **0–6 mm Hg in a spontaneously breathing non-ventilated patient**
  - 'a' wave = atrial contraction
  - 'c' wave = closing and bulging of the tricuspid valve
  - 'x' descent = atrial relaxation
  - 'v' wave = passing filling of atrium
  - 'y' descent = opening of the tricuspid valve
- **CVP waveform analysis.** Catheter sizes are 14–16 gauge. 1.3–1.63 mm in diameter
  - **Zero level set in *mid-axillary line at fourth intercostal space. Reading done at left atrium***
  - **Dominant 'a' wave:** Pulmonary hypertension, tricuspid stenosis, pulmonic stenosis
  - **Cannon 'a' wave:** Complete heart block
  - **Absent 'a' wave:** Atrial fibrillation
  - **Exaggerated 'x' descent:** Pericardial tamponade, constrictive pericarditis
- **PAC waveform:** Pressures and waveform generated while introducing a catheter into the PA
  - 60–110 cm in length and 4–8F in calibre. Balloon inflation volumes range from 0.5–1.5 mL
  - **Lumens:** Four lumens in the catheter
    - **Proximal port:** Terminates 30 cm away from the tip of the catheter in the right atrium. Receives the injectate for cardiac output studies
    - **Thermistor:** A temperature-sensitive wire that terminates *4 cm proximal to tip of the catheter*
    - **Distal port:** At the tip. Allows measurement of PA pressures and measurement of mixed venous SO_2
    - **Balloon:** Inflation/deflation
  - **Pressures:** *PAC shows four types of pressures*
    - **Right atrium:** 20 cm, depicts a CVP waveform. 0–10 mm Hg
    - **Right ventricle:** 30–35 cm. *Pressures:* 15–25 mm Hg
    - **PA:** 40–45 cm, pulmonary artery pressure (PAP): 15–30 mm Hg/ 5–15 mm Hg. Mean PAP: 10–22 mm Hg

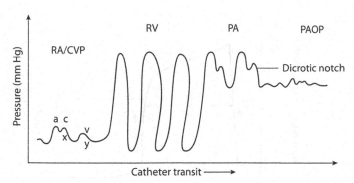

Figure 2.6   PAC with CVP in it.

+ **Wedge position:** 50 cm, pulmonary artery wedge pressure (PAWP): 5–12 mm Hg (approximate LV end-diastolic pressure [LVEDP])
- **PAC data interpretation**
  - **Right heart failure:** high CVP, low cardiac index (CI), high pulmonary vascular resistance (PVR)
  - **Left heart failure:** high pulmonary capillary wedge pressure (PCWP), low CI, high systemic vascular resistance (SVR)
  - **Pericardial tamponade:** high PCWP, high SVR, CVP = PCWP
  - **Hypovolemia:** low CVP, low PCWP, low CI, high SVR
  - **Cardiogenic:** high CVP, high PCWP, low CI, high SVR
  - **Sepsis (distributive):** low CVP, low PCWP, high CI, low SVR

Cardiac action potentials

- **Cardiac myocytes (resting membrane potential [RMP]: –90 mV)**
  - **Phase 0:** Na⁺ influx, upstroke and initial rapid depolarisation
  - **Phase 1:** K⁺ efflux, early rapid repolarisation
  - **Phase 2:** Ca^{2+} influx through slow L-type channels, K⁺ efflux, prolonged plateau phase
  - **Phase 3:** K⁺ efflux, final rapid repolarisation
  - **Phase 4:** 3 Na⁺ out, 2 K⁺ in. Resting membrane potential
- **Pacemaker cells (RMP: –60 mV)**
  - **Phase 0:** Ca^{2+} influx through L-type channels and upstroke
  - **Phase 3:** K⁺ efflux, repolarisation
  - **Phase 4:** Pacemaker potential
    + At –60 mV, funny Na⁺ channels open and Na leaks inside
    + At –50 mV, T-type (transient) Ca^{2+} channels open and there is Ca^{2+} influx

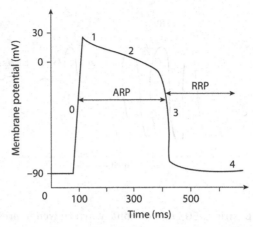

Figure 2.7   Cardiac muscle cell.

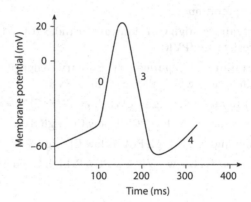

Figure 2.8   Pacemaker node.

Baroreceptors and other cardiac reflexes

- **Baroreceptors:** Nerve endings in the walls of the carotid sinus (chemo-receptors are in the carotid bodies), aorta and heart. **Stretch receptors**
  - *Carotid sinus enlargement of internal carotid artery → ↑ blood Pressure (BP) → ↑ wall stretch → ↑ frequency of impulses discharged → ↓ vasomotor response → ↓ heart rate (HR)*
- **Bainbridge reflex (atrial stretch receptor reflex):** Increase in intravascular volume leads to increase in HR
  - Afferent limb: *Vagus nerves, efferent limb* – Sympathetic nerves to SA node
  - Opposite of baroreceptor reflex
  - After an increase in intravascular pressure, if initial HR is high, baroreceptor reflex happens; if initial HR is low, Bainbridge reflex happens

- **Cushing reflex:** Central reflex due to direct hypoperfusion of vasomotor centre in brainstem. Hypertension and bradycardia
- **Bezold–Jarisch reflex:** Bradycardia and hypotension due to stretching of ventricle wall
  - ○ **Stimulation of inhibitory cardiac receptors by stretching (poorly filled ventricle)**
  - ○ **Cardioprotective effect:** Acts as a positive reflex to vasodilate the coronary arteries during inferoposterior infarction due to coronary vasospasm
  - ○ Parasympathetic reflex to sympathetic overactivity
- **Anrep effect:** Autoregulation method in which myocardial contractility increases with afterload
- **Bowditch effect:** Autoregulation method by which myocardial tension increases with an increase in HR
- **Peripheral chemoreceptor reflex:** Hypoxia and hypercapnia produces increase in BP and transient bradycardia
- **Central chemoreceptor reflex:** Insensitive to hypoxia. Hypercapnia produces an increase in BP and bradycardia
- **Lung volume stretch receptor reflex: Increase in lung volume increases vasodilation**

After an acute blood loss of 1 L, **arteriolar constriction maintains blood pressure. Venoconstriction maintains cardiac output.**

On standing up from lying down, cerebral perfusion pressure is maintained by change in firing of carotid and aortic stretch receptors.

Systemic vs pulmonary circulation

	Systemic circulation (left)	Pulmonary circulation (right)
Distribution of blood	84% (76% in vessels + 8% in heart) About 4500 mL in a 70-kg person	16% About 500 mL in a 70-kg person
Anatomy	• Thick vessels • Abundant thick smooth muscle	• Thin vessels • Minimal smooth muscle • Patency of vessels is dependent upon alveolar pressure

(Continued)

	Systemiac circulation (left)	Pulmonary circulation (right)
Atrial pressures	0–5 mm Hg	6–12 mm Hg
Ventricular pressures	120/10	25/5
Vessels	• Aortic pressure: 120/ 80 mm Hg • Mean arterial pressure (MAP): 100 mm Hg	• Pulmonary pressure: 25/10 • Mean PAP: 15 mm Hg
Circulatory resistance	900–1200 dynes.s/cm^5 $SVR = 80 \times \dfrac{(MAP - CVP)}{CO}$	100–200 dynes.sec/cm^5 PVR = 80 $\times \dfrac{(Mean\ PAP - PAOP)}{CO}$
Response to hypoxia and hypercapnia	Vasodilation	**Vasoconstriction**
Other functions	• NO synthesis • vWF production	• Angiotensin-converting enzyme • Metabolism of serotonin • Metabolism of propofol

Capillaries

- Capillaries contain 6% of the circulating volume
- Surface area of >6000 m^2
- *Capillaries diameter*: 5 μm at arteriolar end and 9 μm at the venous end. *Red blood cell (RBC) diameter:* 7 μm
- Capillaries: Contain a thin layer of epithelial cells and a basement membrane, known as the tunica intima. An incomplete layer of cells in the capillaries that partially encircles the epithelial cells contain pericytes
- Capillaries are of three types
  - Continuous: These capillaries have no perforations
    - Tight junctions between their endothelial cells along with intercellular clefts through which small molecules, like ions, can pass
    - Found in nervous system (blood–brain barrier) and muscles
  - Fenestrated
    - Small openings in their endothelium known as fenestrae or fenestra, which are 80–100 nm in diameter

- ✦ Basement membrane is intact
- ✦ Found in tissues where a large amount of molecular exchange occurs, such as the kidneys, endocrine glands and small intestine
- ○ Sinusoidal: Endothelial linings with multiple fenestrations
  - ✦ 30–40 μm in diameter
  - ✦ Non-existent basal lamina
  - ✦ Found in liver, spleen and lymph nodes

Exercise physiology

- Exercise: Source of energy
  - ○ Immediate energy source: ATP
  - ○ Phosphocreatine system: Stored in skeletal muscle. First 10 s of exercise
- Effect on organ systems
  - ○ Respiratory system
    - ✦ Ventilation increases from resting values of around 5–6 to >200 L/min as both tidal volume and respiratory rate increases. Hence, minute ventilation increases a maximum of 30–35 times during exercise
    - ✦ Oxygen consumption increases from 250–5000 mL/min in an endurance athlete
    - ✦ Oxyhaemoglobin dissociation curve is shifted to the right
  - ○ Cardiovascular system
    - ✦ HR and SV increase to about 90% of their maximum values during strenuous exercise in trained athletes (HR about 180/min and SV 160 mL)
    - ✦ ↑ BP (systolic BP [SBP] > diastolic BP [DBP])
    - ✦ Coronary blood flow increases three times from 250–750 mL/min
    - ✦ Lactate increases from 1–10 mmol/L
  - ○ Central nervous system
    - ✦ Cerebral blood flow remains unchanged at 750 mL/min
    - ✦ Activation of sympathetic nervous systems
  - ○ Skeletal muscle system
    - ✦ Resting blood flow to muscle is usually 1200 mL/min but increases to nearly 12,500 mL/min during maximal exercise due to β_2 sympathetic stimulation
    - ✦ Main reason is relaxation of skeletal muscle precapillary sphincters

- ○ Other systems
  - ◆ Blood supply to viscera decreases from 1400 to 600 mL/min
  - ◆ Blood supply to skin increases from 500 mL/min to 1900 mL/min
  - ◆ Temperature increases because of hypermetabolic muscles

Post-anaesthetic shivering can also increase oxygen consumption by up to 3–5 times.

Valsalva manoeuvre

- • **Valsalva manoeuvre:** Expiration against a closed glottis. Pressure of 40 mm Hg held for 10 s
- • Phases

  1. **Phase I:** Acute increase in intrathoracic pressure compresses thoracic veins. Venous return is increased to left atrium. This causes an **increase in BP** with a compensatory reduction in HR
  2. **Phase II:** Sustained increase in intrathoracic pressure impedes further venous return. This leads to lowering BP, which causes **reflex tachycardia**
  3. **Phase III:** Intrathoracic pressure is released in this stage. Venous return pools in the pulmonary vessels due to fall in intrathoracic pressure, thus, BP decreases. HR stays high

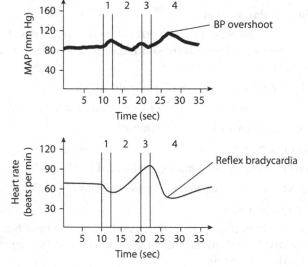

Figure 2.9   Valsalva manoeuvre.

4. **Phase IV:** The raised HR restores BP, and SBP exceeds the resting value. This rise in BP again leads to reflex bradycardia. All parameters ultimately return to normal

- Pathologies

  - **Diabetes:** Autonomic neuropathy blunts baroreceptor activation. Hence, BP drops excessively during phase II. Overshoot of phase IV is absent

  - **Congestive heart failure:** Square wave response. No increase in BP or HR when intrathoracic pressure is released

Cardiopulmonary exercise testing

- **CPET:** Non-invasive, objective and repeatable assessment of combined pulmonary and cardiac function
- **Mechanism:** Electromagnetically braked cycle ergometer is used
  - **Duration of test: 10 min**
  - Measurements are taken
    - At rest
    - During unloaded cycling (pedalling without any resistance)
    - Pedalling against a continuously increasing resistance (increasing work at a predetermined ramp rate)
    - Recovery phase immediately after exercise
- **Anaerobic threshold (AT):** It marks the onset of anaerobic metabolism as a result of inadequate oxygen delivery
  - An AT of at least 11 mL/kg/min is required to safely undertake major surgery
- **Peak O_2 consumption (Peak VO_2):** Maximum VO_2 that is measured at the point that exercise is terminated
  - Peak VO_2 less than 15 mL O_2 kg/min means greater risk of perioperative complication
- **Ventilatory equivalent (V_E/VCO_2):** Amount in litres you have to breathe to get rid of 1 L CO_2 each minute. Minute ventilation/volume of CO_2 exhaled
  - VE/VCO$_2$ at <34 means fit patient
- **Metabolic equivalent (MET):** 1 MET is defined as the energy you use when you're resting or sitting still. 1 MET = 3.5 mL O_2/kg/min
- The ability to climb more than five flights of stairs correlates with a VO_2 peak of >20 mL/kg/min, whilst those able to climb less than one flight of stairs correlates with a VO_2 peak of <10 mL/kg/min[3]

- Functional walk tests: Other tests for checking functional capacity
  - 6-min walk test (6MWT): It measures how far subjects can walk along a flat corridor, turning around cones at each end, at normal pace, in 6 min
    - Healthy subjects can walk around 500–600 m
  - Incremental shuttle walk test (ISWT): Walking conducted along a 10-m course. The walking speed increases every minute until the patient is too breathless to continue. The result is given as the total distance achieved

Pacemakers

- **Pacemakers:** Devices that detect the slow/abnormal electrical activity of the heart and stimulate it to contract at a faster rate
- **Classification:** North American Society of Pacing and Electrophysiology (NASPE) and the British Pacing and Electrophysiology Group (BPEG) in 2002

I	II	III	IV	V
Chambers paced	Chambers sensed	Response to sensing	Rate modulation	Multisite pacing
0 = None	0 = None	0 = None	0 = None	0 = None
A = Atrium	A = Atrium	I = Inhibited	R = Rate modulation	A = Atrium
V = Ventricle	V = Ventricle	T = Triggered		V = Ventricle
D = Dual (A+V)	D = Dual (A+V)	D = Dual (A+V)		D = Dual (A+V)

- **I:** Indicates that a sensed event inhibits the output pulse
- **T:** Indicates that an output pulse is triggered in response to a sensed event
- **R:** R in the fourth position indicates that the pacemaker has rate modulation and incorporates a sensor to adjust its programmed paced HR in response to patient activity like exercise
- **Asynchronous pacing modes:** Used for patients who are undergoing a surgical procedure, especially if the patient is pacemaker dependent
  - **Electrocautery could be sensed by the pacemaker and misinterpreted as native cardiac activity, thereby inhibiting pacing output producing bradycardia or asystole**
  - Prior to surgery, the pacemaker could be reprogrammed to an asynchronous mode by a technician

- o Magnet over pacemakers: No longer recommended. They turn pacemaker into asynchronous mode and are only applicable to older non-reprogrammable pacemakers
- Decision if a device needs to be altered prior to surgery

  - o Anticipated amount of electromagnetic interference (EMI)
  - o Type of device (pacemaker, implantable cardioverter defibrillator [ICD] or cardiac resynchronisation therapy [CRT])
  - o Pacemaker dependency
  - o Rate adaptive features
- If surgery is not around the pacemaker and use of diathermy is minimal, then there is no need to alter the pacemaker
- If a rate-modulated pacemaker used, then this feature should be deactivated prior to theatre

Myocardial Infarction

- Myocardial Infarction (MI) is defined as myocardial necrosis in a clinical setting consistent with myocardial ischemia. These conditions include a rise of cardiac markers (cardiac troponins [cTn]) above the 99th percentile of the upper reference limit plus at least one of the following:
  - o Symptoms of ischemia
  - o ECG changes indicative of new ischemia, significant ST/T changes or left bundle branch block
  - o Development of pathologic Q waves
  - o Imaging evidence of new loss of myocardium or new regional wall motion abnormality
  - o Angiography or autopsy evidence of intracoronary thrombus
- MI can be classified into five types based on aetiology and circumstances
  - o Type 1: Spontaneous MI caused by ischemia due to a primary coronary event (e.g., plaque rupture, erosion, coronary dissection)
  - o Type 2: Ischemia due to ischemic imbalance, i.e., increased oxygen demand (e.g., hypertension), or decreased supply (e.g., coronary artery spasm, embolism)
  - o Type 3: Related to sudden unexpected cardiac death
  - o Type 4a: Associated with percutaneous coronary intervention (PCI)
  - o Type 4b: Associated with documented stent thrombosis
  - o Type 5: Associated with coronary artery bypass grafting (CABG)

- ECG changes and coronary arteries

Infarct	Changes in ECG	ECG leads	Artery involved
Anterior	ST elevation	V1, V2, V3, V4	Left anterior descending (LAD)
Inferior	ST elevation	II, III, aVF	Right coronary artery (RCA)
Lateral	ST elevation	I, aVL, V5, V6	Left circumflex (LCX)
Posterior	ST depression, Tall R wave	V1, V2	RCA or LCX

\# LV failure: Hypotension, pulmonary oedema

\# Right ventricular failure: High CVP, pedal oedema

Central Nervous System

3

Cerebral circulation

- **Normal cerebral blood flow (CBF):** 15% of cardiac output = 750 mL/min = 50 mL/100 g/min
  - **White matter:** 20 mL/100 g/min
  - **Grey matter:** 70 mL/100 g/min
- **Cerebral arterial supply:** Two-thirds supplied by internal carotid arteries (ICAs). One-third supplied by vertebral arteries. Basilar arteries are formed by joining two vertebral arteries
  - **ICA:** Arises from common carotid arteries
  - **Anterior cerebral artery:** Terminal branch of the ICA
  - **Middle cerebral artery:** Terminal branch of the ICA. Technically not a part of circle of Willis.
  - **Anterior communicating artery (ACOM):** Joins the right and left anterior cerebral arteries
  - **Posterior cerebral artery:** These vessels arise from bifurcation of the basilar artery
  - **Posterior communicating artery (PCOM):** It is a branch of the ICA. Joins the posterior cerebral artery to the ICA

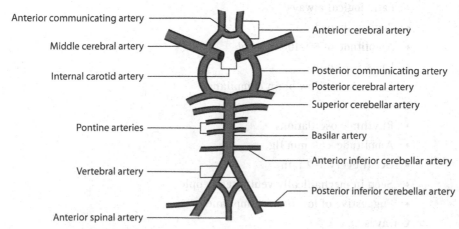

Anterior communicating artery
Middle cerebral artery
Internal carotid artery
Pontine arteries
Vertebral artery
Anterior spinal artery

Anterior cerebral artery
Posterior communicating artery
Posterior cerebral artery
Superior cerebellar artery
Basilar artery
Anterior inferior cerebellar artery
Posterior inferior cerebellar artery

Figure 3.1 Circle of Willis.

DOI: 10.1201/9781003390244-4

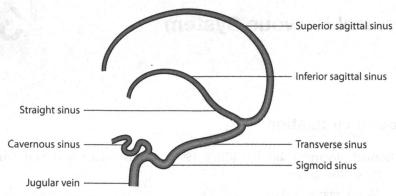

Figure 3.2 Venous drainage.

Intracranial pressure waves

- Intracranial pressure (ICP)waves have three characteristic peaks due to cardiac cycle
  - **P1:** Percussive wave due to arterial pulsation
  - **P2:** Tidal wave due to both arterial pulsation and resistance from brain parenchyma
  - **P3:** Dicrotic wave due to closure of aortic valve
- Normal order of height is P1 > P2 > P3. If P2 is highest, this indicates potential raised ICP
- Decrease in brain compliance causes pathological waves. Lundberg classified them in three patterns
  - **A waves**
    - Pathological always
    - Plateau shaped
    - Amplitude of 50–100 mm Hg
    - Lasts 2–20 min
    - Suggestive of low brain compliance
  - **B waves**
    - Rhythmic oscillations
    - Amplitude <50 mm Hg
    - Occur every 1–2 min
    - Seen in mechanically ventilated people
    - Suggestive of low brain compliance
  - **C waves**
    - Non-pathological

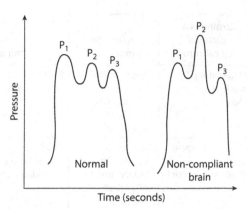

Figure 3.3   ICP waveform.

- ◆ Rhythmic oscillations
- ◆ Amplitude <20 mm Hg
- ◆ Occur every 4–8 min
- ◆ Less used clinically
- • Pressures greater than 20 mm Hg usually represent the threshold to treat raised ICP
  - ○ Most common ICP monitoring indication is severe traumatic brain injury (TBI)
  - ○ Monitors are usually inserted at Kocher's point which is an entry point through the frontal bone for an intraventricular catheter to cerebro-spinal fluid (CSF)
- • Most common ICP monitoring indication is severe Traumatic brain injury (TBI)

Cranial nerves

Cranial nerve	Brainstem nucleus/ Cerebrum	Structures innervated	Functions	Foramina
Olfactory	- Primary olfactory cortex (POC) located in temporal lobe - Amygdala	Olfactory epithelium	Olfaction	Cribriform plate
Optic	- Primary visual cortex in occipital lobe	Olfactory epithelium	Vision	Optic canal

(Continued)

Cranial nerve	Brainstem nucleus/ Cerebrum	Structures innervated	Functions	Foramina
Oculomotor (Midbrain)	Oculomotor nucleus (Motor)	- Superior/middle/ inferior rectus. Inferior oblique - Levator palpebrae	Eyeball movements	Superior orbital fissure
	Edinger–Westphal nucleus (Parasympathetic)	Pupillary constrictor and ciliary muscle of eyeball via the ciliary ganglion	Pupillary constriction and accommodation	
Trochlear (Midbrain)	Trochlear nucleus (Motor)	Superior oblique muscle	Eyeball movement	Superior orbital fissure
Trigeminal (Pons)	Motor	- Masseter, Temporal, medial and lateral pterygoids - Tensor veli palatini, mylohyoid, anterior belly of digastric and tensor tympani	- Mastication - Tension of tympanic membrane	- Superior orbital fissure (Ophthalmic V_1) (Sensory) - Foramen rotundum (Maxillary V_2) (Sensory) - Foramen ovale (Mandibular V_3) (Mixed)
	Primary sensory	Face and oral cavity	Touch	
	Mesencephalic (Sensory)	Periodontium and the muscles of mastication in the jaw (Jaw jerk reflex)	Proprioception	
	Spinal tract (Sensory)	Face and oral cavity	Pain and temperature	
Abducens (Pons)	Abducens nucleus (Motor)	Lateral rectus muscle	Eyeball movement	Superior orbital fissure
Facial (Pons)	Nucleus solitarius (Sensory)	**Anterior two-thirds of tongue**	Taste	Internal acoustic meatus
	Facial motor nucleus	Muscles of facial expression	Facial movement	
		Stapedius muscle	Tension of ossicles	

(*Continued*)

Cranial nerve	Brainstem nucleus/ Cerebrum	Structures innervated	Functions	Foramina
Facial (Pons) (Cont'd)	Superior salivatory nucleus (Parasympathetic)	Salivary and lacrimal glands via submandibular and pterygopalatine ganglia	Salivation and lacrimation	
Vestibulocochlear (Pons)	Vestibular (Sensory)	Vestibular apparatus	Proprioception of head and balance	Internal acoustic meatus
	Cochlea (Sensory)	Cochlea	Hearing	
Glossopharyngeal (Medulla)	Spinal tract nucleus of trigeminal via petrosal ganglion (Sensory)	Eustachian tube and middle ear	General sensation	Jugular foramen
	Rostral part of Nucleus solitarius (Sensory)	Pharynx and posterior one-third of tongue	Taste	
	Caudal part of nucleus solitarius (Sensory)	Carotid body	Chemoreception and baroreception	
	Nucleus ambiguous (Motor)	Stylopharyngeus	Swallowing	
	Inferior salivatory nucleus (Parasympathetic)	Salivary glands via otic ganglion	Salivation	
Vagus (Medulla)	Spinal trigeminal nucleus via nodose ganglion (Sensory)	Pharynx, larynx, oesophagus till colon	General sensation	Jugular foramen
	Rostral part of nucleus solitarius (Sensory)	Epiglottis	Taste sensation	
	Caudal part of nucleus solitarius (Sensory)	Carotid body	Chemoreception and baroreception	
	Nucleus ambiguous (Motor)	- Soft palate, larynx, pharynx and upper oesophagus (Motor) - Cardiac parasympathetic	- Speech and swallowing - Preganglionic parasympathetic neurons that innervate the heart	

(Continued)

Cranial nerve	Brainstem nucleus/ Cerebrum	Structures innervated	Functions	Foramina
Vagus (Medulla) (*Cont'd*)	Dorsal motor nucleus (Parasympathetic)	Cardiac, lung and gastrointestinal systems	Visceral parasympathetic system	
Spinal accessory (Medulla)	Nucleus ambiguous (Motor) Spinal accessory nucleus (Motor)	Sternomastoid and trapezius	Movement of head and shoulders	Jugular foramen
Hypoglossal (Medulla)	Hypoglossal nucleus (Motor)	Intrinsic and extrinsic muscles of tongue	Movement of tongue	Hypoglossal canal

- **Tongue:** Sensory supply
  - General sensation of the anterior two-thirds is supplied by the **trigeminal nerve** (cranial nerve [CN] V). The **lingual nerve** is a branch of the **mandibular nerve** (CN V3)
  - Taste in the anterior two-thirds is supplied from the **facial nerve** (CN VII)
  - The posterior one-third of the tongue is slightly easier. Both touch and taste are supplied by the **glossopharyngeal nerve** (CN IX)

Cerebral blood flow

- Cerebral perfusion pressure (CPP) = mean arterial pressure (MAP) − (ICP + central venous pressure [CVP]). Maintain CPP >70 mm Hg
- ICP: Pressure exerted by CSF inside the skull and on the brain tissue
  - **Normal:** 10–15 mm Hg
  - **Supine:** 7–15 mm Hg
  - **Elevated:** Greater than 20 mm Hg
- **Monro–Kellie doctrine:** The skull is a rigid box with a constant volume. Increase in volume of one of the contents is compensated by a reduction in volume of another
  - **Brain** 80%, CSF 10%, blood 10%
- *CBF* = 50 mL/100g/min. CBF is autoregulated between a MAP of about 50 to 150 mm Hg

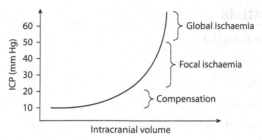

Figure 3.4   Monro–Kellie doctrine.

- **Autoregulation of CBF**
  - ○ Intrinsic control:
    1. **Metabolic:** H^+, K^+, adenosine, nitric oxide (NO) and CO_2 causes vasodilation
    2. Myogenic
  - ○ Extrinsic control: *Neurogenic or autonomic nervous system (ANS):* Sympathetic nervous system (SNS) and parasympathetic nervous system (PNS)
- *Cerebral metabolic requirement for oxygen (CMRO₂):* Falls by 7% per 1°C decrease in body temperature
- Factors increasing CBF. CBF is measured by the **Kety–Schmidt method**
  - ○ Hypercapnia (CBF increases linearly between a $PaCO_2$ of 2.7 kPa and 10.7 kPa)
  - ○ Hypoxia (unaffected until 7 kPa, then doubles at PaO_2 of 4 kPa)
  - ○ Acidosis
  - ○ Volatile anaesthetics
  - ○ Ketamine
- **Factors decreasing CBF**
  - ○ Hypocapnia
  - ○ Hypothermia
  - ○ All intravenous induction agents except ketamine

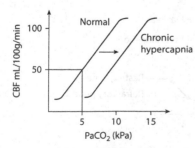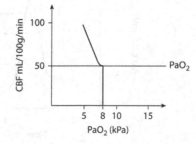

Figure 3.5   Effects of ventilation on CBF.

Action potentials

Resting membrane potential

- Neuron: –70 mV
- Myocyte: –90 mV
- SA node: –60 mV
- Purkinje fibre: –90 mV
- Ventricle: –90 mV

	Absolute refractive period	Relative refractive period
Neuron	1 ms	2–3 ms
Cardiac muscle	200 ms	100 ms

Nernst equation: Used to calculate the membrane potential for a single ion assuming that the cell membrane is completely permeable to that ion: Na^+ +50 mV, Cl^- –70 mV, K^+ –90 mV.

Goldman equation: Resting membrane potential can be more precisely quantified by considering all the ionic permeabilities using the Goldman equation.

Fibre type	Function	Diameter (µm)	Conduction velocity (m/s)
Aα	Somatic motor and proprioception	12–20	70–120
Aβ	Touch and pressure	5–12	50–70
Aγ	Motor fibres to muscle spindles	3–6	30–50
Aδ	Pain, temperature and touch	2–5	<30
B	Myelinated pre-ganglionic autonomic fibres	1–3	<15
C	Unmyelinated post-ganglionic autonomic fibres, pain and temperature	1	1

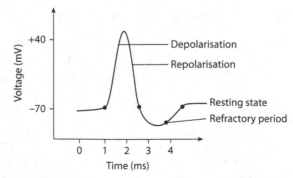

Figure 3.6 Action potential of a nerve.

Increasing the extracellular concentration of potassium ions would have the greatest effect in making the resting membrane potential less negative.

Na-K ATPase pump is the most important mechanism in maintaining the magnitude of the resting membrane potential.

Cerebrospinal Fluid

- Volume of CSF: 150 mL
- CSF is production @ 0.4 mL/min or 500 mL/day
- Produced by the choroid plexus and absorbed by arachnoid villi
- **Passage:** Flows from the lateral ventricle via the foramen of Munro to the third ventricle. From the third ventricle via the aqueduct of Sylvius to the fourth ventricle. From the fourth ventricle CSF leaves via the single foramen of Magendie or two foramina of Luschka
- **Specific gravity:** 1.006–1.007, clear colourless
- **Lymphocytes:** 0–5/mm^3 with nil polymorphs
- **Bacterial meningitis:** Predominantly polymorphs increased with decreased CSF to plasma glucose
- **Viral meningitis:** Predominantly lymphocytes increased with usually normal CSF glucose

Parameter	CSF	Blood
pH	7.33	7.40
Osmolarity	295 mOsm/L	295 mOsm/L
Sodium	144–152 mmol/L	135–145 mmol/L
Chloride	**123–128 mmol/L**	95–105 mmol/L
Potassium	2–3 mmol/L	3.5–5 mmol/L
Calcium	1.1–1.3 mmol/L	2.2–2.6 mmol/L
Urea	2–7 mmol/L	2.5–6.5 mmol/L
Glucose	**2.5–4.5 mmol/L**	3–5 mmol/L
Protein	200–400 mg/L (0.5% of plasma)	60–80 g/L

- Lack of protein in CSF gives it reduced buffering capacity

Spinal cord

- Spinal cord: From foramen magnum to L1 in adults and until L3 at birth
  - There are 31 pairs of spinal nerves, 8 pairs of cervical, 12 pairs of thoracic, 5 pairs of lumbar, 5 pairs of sacral and one pair of coccygeal nerve

- o *Grey matter:* Cell bodies of neurons and unmyelinated axons
- o *White matter:* Surrounds grey matter, ascending and descending neuron tracts
- **Arterial supply:** Single anterior spinal artery and two posterior spinal arteries
  - o Anterior spinal artery formed at the level of foramen magnum by coming together of the two branches of the vertebral arteries. Anterior two-thirds of cord is supplied
  - o Posterior spinal artery given by posterior inferior cerebellar arteries. The posterior one-third of cord is supplied
  - o Radicular branches arise from local arteries and supply the spinal cord. Radicularis magna or artery of Adamkiewicz supplies lower thoracic and higher lumbar areas between T8 and L3
- **Ascending tracts:** Sensory axons
  - o **Dorsal column:** *Fine touch, proprioception and vibration sense* from ipsilateral side of the body
    - • **Gracile fasciculus:** Medially and from lower half of body
    - • **Cuneate fasciculus:** Laterally and from upper part of body
  - o **Lateral spinothalamic tracts:** Pain and temperature from the contralateral side of the body
  - o **Anterior spinothalamic tracts:** Crude touch and pressure from the contralateral side of the body
  - o **Spinocerebellar tracts:** Anterior and posterior tracts. Proprioception from ipsilateral side of the body to the cerebellum
  - o **Spinotectal tract:** Sensory information to the brainstem
- **Descending tracts:** Motor axons
  - o **Anterior and lateral corticospinal tracts:** Pyramidal tract. To contralateral side of the body. Innervates muscle
  - o **Extrapyramidal tracts:** Rubrospinal, tectospinal, vestibulospinal tracts. Control of posture and muscle tone
- **Brown–Sequard syndrome:** Hemisection of spinal cord
  - o Loss of fine touch on the same side of body
  - o Loss of proprioception and vibration sense on the same side of the body
  - o Loss of pain and temperature on the contralateral side of the body
  - o Muscle weakness on the same side
- **Syringomyelia:** Central cord expands
  - o Loss of pain and temperature at level of syrinx

- o Preservation of the two-point discrimination, proprioception and vibration sensation
- **Lateral medullary syndrome:** Lateral medulla infarction due to occlusion of the posterior inferior cerebellar artery
  - o Loss of pain sensation on the contralateral side of the body and same side of the face
- **Acute spinal cord injury:** Symptoms depend on level of body injured
  - o CVS: *Above T6* – 'Neurogenic shock' due to disruption of sympathetic nervous outflow
    - *Above T1:* Bradycardia due to disruption of cardio acceleratory fibres
  - o **Respiratory:** *Above T8* – Intercostal muscle paralysis
    - **At level of C3:** Diaphragm paralysis
  - o **Nervous system:** *Initially, flaccid paralysis* and loss of reflexes below the level of spinal cord lesion known as *spinal shock*. Bladder becomes atonic and priapism happens
    - Spastic paralysis over the next 3 weeks. Extensor response
  - o **Gastrointestinal system:** Unopposed parasympathetic input due to disruption of sympathetic fibres
    - Delayed gastric emptying, gastric ulceration, paralytic ileus and constipation
- **Cauda equina syndrome:** Lesion below the level of L2 compresses the nerve roots rather than the spinal cord
  - o Severe leg weakness with partially preserved sensation
  - o Saddle anaesthesia with numbness around anus, buttocks and perineum
  - o Urinary retention

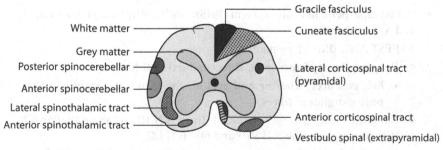

Figure 3.7   Cross section of spinal cord.

Autonomic nervous system

- ANS: Involved in the involuntary control of homeostasis and mounting stress response. Divided into sympathetic and PNSs
- SNS: Lateral horns of the spinal cords from T1 to L2 (thoracolumbar)
  - FLIGHT OR FIGHT response
  - *Preganglionic fibres:* Short, slow conducting B fibres
    - Releases acetylcholine and acts on the nicotinic receptors of the post-ganglionic fibres
  - *Ganglia:* Close to spinal cord
    - Paravertebral ganglia: Run on either side of vertebra from base of skull to coccyx
      1. Cervical: Superior, middle and inferior. Inferior cervical ganglion fuses with first thoracic ganglion to form stellate ganglion
      2. Thoracic: 12 ganglia, one for each segment. T1–T5 supplies cardiac plexus
      3. Lumbar: Branches given to coeliac plexus
      4. Pelvis: Sacral ganglia
    - Prevertebral ganglia: Anterior to major arteries
      1. Coeliac plexus
      2. Superior mesenteric
      3. Inferior mesenteric
    - White rami communicantes connect SNS pre-ganglionic fibres to paravertebral ganglia
  - *Post-ganglionic fibres:* Long, slow conducting unmyelinated C fibres
    - Release noradrenaline normally at all times except acetylcholine when innervating sweat glands on cholinergic muscarinic receptors
    - Adrenal medulla acts as a specialised post-ganglionic fibre and releases adrenaline (80%) and noradrenaline (20%)
    - Grey rami communicantes connect SNS ganglia to spinal nerves
- Parasympathetic nervous system (PNS): CN III, VII, IX and X and S_2, S_3 and S_4 sacral nerves
  - REST AND DIGEST response
  - *Pre-ganglionic fibres:* Long, slow conducting B fibres
    - Releases acetylcholine and acts on the nicotinic receptors of the post-ganglionic fibres
  - *Ganglia:* Close to target tissues. Ciliary (CN III), submandibular (CN VII), pterygopalatine (CN VII) and otic (CN IX)
  - *Post-ganglionic fibres:* Short, slow conducting unmyelinated C fibres
    - Release acetylcholine normally at all times and acts on cholinergic muscarinic receptor

Target organ/ Tissues		Sympathetic nervous system		Parasympathetic nervous system
Blood vessels	α_1 α_2 β_2	Vasoconstriction Presynaptic inhibition of noradrenaline release Vasodilation	M3	Vasodilatation
Heart	β_1	Positive chronotropy and inotropy	M2	Negative chronotropy and inotropy
Bronchi	β_2	Bronchodilation	M3	Bronchoconstriction
Pupils	α_1	Pupil dilatation	M3	Pupillary constriction
Ciliary muscles	β_2 β_2	Ciliary muscle relaxation Aqueous humour production	M3	Ciliary muscle contraction
Gut smooth muscles	α_2, β_2	Relaxes smooth muscles of GIT	M3	Increases peristalsis
GI tract sphincters	α_1	Contraction of GI tract sphincters	M3	Relaxation of sphincters except lower oesophagus
			M1	Increased secretion of glands except pancreas
Liver	α_1, β_2 $\alpha1$, $\beta1$, β_3 α_2	Glycogenolysis Lipolysis Inhibition of lipolysis	M3	Constriction of biliary tract
Kidney	β_1, β_2	Renin release from juxtaglomerular apparatus (JGA)		
Urinary tract	α_1 β_2	Contraction of detrusor Detrusor relaxation, sphincter contraction (urinary retention)	M3	Detrusor contraction, sphincter relaxation (micturition)
Uterus	α_1 β_2	Contraction Relaxation		
Platelets	α_2	Platelet aggregation		
Hair follicles	α_1	Piloerection		
Salivary gland	α_1	Thick viscous secretion		

Pain

- **Pain:** An unpleasant sensory and emotional experience associated with actual or potential tissue damage
- **Hyperalgesia:** Increased response to painful stimuli
- **Allodynia:** Pain resulting from normally non-painful tactile stimuli
- **Peripheral sensory transmission:** From stimuli to spinal cords
  - Classification of nerves that carry sensory information
    - Aβ fibres: Large in diameter and highly myelinated
      - Quick conduction of action potentials
      - Light touch and tactile information
    - Aδ fibres: Smaller in diameter and thinly myelinated
      - Thermal and mechanical stimuli
    - C fibres: Smallest in diameter and unmyelinated
      - Painful stimuli
  - Nociceptors: Pain receptors are unmyelinated nerve endings
  - Tissue injury leads to release of prostaglandins (**non-steroidal anti-inflammatory drugs [NSAIDs]**), bradykinin, histamine, serotonin, acetylcholine, H⁺ and K⁺ ions, which stimulate nociceptors
- **Sensory transmission at dorsal horn**
  - The cell bodies of Aβ, Aδ and C fibres lie in the dorsal root ganglia
  - The fibres terminate in dorsal horn and synapse with secondary afferent neurons in an area known as Rexed laminae
  - Aδ and C fibres terminate in laminae I–II of the dorsal horn
  - Aβ fibres terminate in laminae III–VI of the dorsal horn
  - **Substantia gelatinosa:** Rexed lamina II where C fibres terminate. Involved in gate control of pain
- **Mechanisms of modulation of nociceptive transmission at spinal cord**
  - Glutamate is an excitatory neurotransmitter. Released by primary afferent nerves for transmission in dorsal horn
  - Glutamate acts on three types of receptors present on secondary afferent neurons
    - α-amino-3-hydroxy 5-methyl-4-isoxazeloproprionic acid *(AMPA)* receptor: Fast initial activation
    - N-methyl-D-aspartate *(NMDA) receptors:* Repetitive stimulation of C fibres. Amplification and prolongation of the response
      - Hyperalgesia and allodynia are because of NMDA receptors. Antagonists of NMDA receptors give pain relief (ketamine)

- Winding up: The pain signal that comes into the central nervous system becomes stronger and longer lasting because of NMDA receptors
  - G-protein-coupled metabotropic receptors (mGluR)
- Inhibitory neurotransmitters are **enkephalins (opioids)** and gamma-aminobutyric acid (GABA)
- Spinal projections to brain
  - At lamina I, primary afferent neurons synapse with second-order neurons that have neurokinin 1 (NK1) receptors
    - Substance P is released from afferent nociceptive peripheral nerves
    - NK1 positive cells project in the brain to areas such as thalamus, periaqueductal grey (PAG) and parabrachial (PB) areas
    - These cells also project into brainstem areas with rostral ventromedial medulla (RVM), which has descending projections back to the dorsal horn
  - Lamina III–VI neurons project mainly to the thalamus
    - From the thalamus, nociceptive information is transmitted to cortical regions like primary and secondary somatosensory cortices and insular, anterior cingulate and prefrontal cortices
- **Brainstem modulation of dorsal horn pathways**
  - Both facilitatory and inhibitory in nature
  - Descending facilitatory RVM pathways cause maintenance of nerve injury-induced pain
    - **5-HT$_3$** receptors exert this effect. Antagonists at 5-HT$_3$ receptors help in pain relief (**tramadol, gabapentin**)
  - Descending inhibitory involves the release of norepinephrine in spinal cord from brainstem nuclei such as **locus coeruleus (LC)**
    - Acts on α_2 adrenoreceptor receptors (**clonidine**)
- **Gate control theory of pain:** Pain transmission from primary afferents to secondary afferents is gated by interneurons in the substantia gelatinosa
  - Opening of gate and ↑ transmission of pain
    - Presynaptic release of substance P by C fibres
    - Postsynaptic by Aδ fibres as they inhibit the action of enkephalinergic interneurons (**low-frequency transcutaneous electrical nerve stimulation [TENS]**)
  - Closure of gate and ↓ transmission of pain
    - Presynaptic inhibition of C fibres by release of GABA by Aβ fibres
    - Postsynaptic by descending inhibitory fibres as they activate the action of enkephalinergic interneurons (**high-frequency TENS**)

Eye

- **Bony orbit:** Globe axial length is 24 mm, >26 mm is myopic
  - **Roof:** Orbital plate of the frontal bone
  - **Floor:** Zygoma and maxilla
  - **Medial wall:** Parts of maxilla, lacrimal bone, ethmoid, sphenoid
  - **Lateral wall:** Zygoma, greater wing of the sphenoid
- **Aqueous humour:** Clear gelatinous fluid within the anterior and posterior chambers of the eye
  - Production is 2 mL/day
  - Produced by the ciliary processes of the ciliary body and secreted into the posterior chamber
  - Flows between iris and lens and into the anterior chamber through the pupil
  - Exits the anterior chamber via the trabecular meshwork at the iridocorneal angle into the canal of Schlemm (a sinus that drains into anterior ciliary veins that drain into superior ophthalmic vein and then into the cavernous sinus)
  - Some exit through the uveoscleral route and get absorbed into the ciliary muscle
- **Intraocular pressure (IOP):** Normal is 10–25 mm Hg
  - Factors affecting IOP
    - Choroidal blood flow, which is autoregulated by hypoxia, hypercarbia, coughing and straining
    - Aqueous humour production and drainage (pupil dilatation decreases drainage)
    - **Extraocular muscle tone:** All intravenous induction agents except ketamine lower IOP. Volatiles lower IOP. N_2O can interact with SF6 (sulphur hexafluoride) to increase volume of gas and cause increased IOP. Non-depolarising muscle relaxants lower IOP but suxamethonium causes slight rise in IOP
  - Drugs affecting IOP
    - **Reduce aqueous humour production:** Beta-blockers, carbonic anhydrase inhibitors
    - **Improve aqueous humour drainage:** Prostaglandins, miotic drugs, e.g., pilocarpine
- **Nerve supply to the eye**
  - **Sensory:** Ophthalmic division of trigeminal (nasociliary and long ciliary) nerve
    - Optic nerve for vision

- o Motor to extraocular muscle: $LR_6(SO_4)_3$
  - ◆ Lateral rectus supplied by abducens nerve; superior oblique by trochlear nerve and the rest of the muscles by oculomotor nerve
- **Mydriasis:** Sympathetic innervation goes through superior cervical ganglion and passes through long ciliary nerves (CN V_1) or ciliary ganglion (without synapse) via the short ciliary nerves to supply the dilator pupillae (radial fibres of the iris)
  - o **Drugs:** Anticholinergic (atropine, cyclopentolate, tropicamide), sympathomimetics (e.g., topical phenylephrine), central (ketamine)
- **Miosis:** Parasympathetic innervation originates from Edinger–Westphal nucleus in the midbrain. Goes through the oculomotor nerve to the ciliary ganglion (with synapse) via the short ciliary nerves to cause contraction of sphincter pupillae (circular fibres of the iris) and contraction of the ciliary muscles (thickens the lens to allow focus on near objects to cause accommodation)
  - o **Drugs:** Parasympathomimetics (pilocarpine), opioids, central action (e.g., antipsychotics)
- **Pupillary light reflex:** Constriction of the pupil in response to light, thereby adjusting the amount of light that reaches the retina
  - o Optic nerve → pretectal nucleus of midbrain → Edinger–Westphal nucleus → ciliary ganglion → sphincter pupillae
- **Corneal Reflex:** Touching the cornea causes blinking
  - o **Afferent:** Nasociliary branch of CN V_1 (trigeminal nerve)
  - o **Efferent:** Temporal and zygomatic branches of CN VII (facial nerve)
- **Oculocardiac reflex/Aschner reflex:** Bradycardia or asystole observed as a result of traction on the extraocular muscles
  - o **Afferent:** Stretch receptors on ocular tissues, via the long and short ciliary nerves to ciliary ganglion. From here, impulses are transported via the ophthalmic division of the trigeminal nerve to the gasserian ganglion, followed by the trigeminal nucleus
  - o **Efferent:** Through vagus nerve to sinoatrial (SA) node causing bradycardia
- **Ptosis:** Injury to CN III as it supplies the levator palpebrae superioris
  - o Injury to cervical sympathetic chain due to loss of superior tarsal muscle
- **Anaesthesia for eye surgery**
  - o **Topical:** Topical amethocaine 0.5%, oxybuprocaine 0.4%, proxymetacaine 0.5%
    - ◆ Lack of akinesia of eye and eyelids

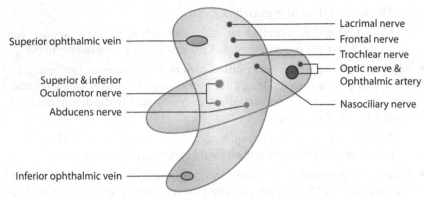

Figure 3.8 Orbit.

- o **Retrobulbar block:** Single injection using a 25-mm needle, 3–4 mL of anaesthetic given at the junction of lateral and middle thirds of the orbital margin in the inferotemporant quadrant
  - ◆ **Complications:** Retrobulbar haemorrhage, penetration of the globe, damage to the optic nerve or ophthalmic vessels, central spread of local anaesthetic
- o **Peribulbar block:** Total 8–10 mL of anaesthetic given via two injections. Less complications compared with retrobulbar block
  - ◆ 5 mL via inferotemporal injection and 4 mL via superonasal injection
- o **Sub-tenon block:** Dissection done using Westcott scissors in the inferomedial quadrant of the globe. Find the sub-tenon plane to dissect down to bare sclera. A specially designed blunt cannula to inject 3–4 mL of anaesthetic is given

Nose

- • **Nose:** Fibres of the olfactory nerve (CN I) pass through the cribriform plate of the ethmoid bone to synapse directly with cells in the olfactory bulb
- • **Boundaries of nasal cavity**
  - o **Roof:** Nasal, frontal, sphenoid and cribriform plate of ethmoid
  - o **Floor:** Maxillary anteriorly and palatine bone posteriorly
  - o **Medial wall:** Upper part is the perpendicular plate of ethmoid and vomer. Lower part is cartilaginous
  - o **Lateral wall:** Ethmoid above it
    - ◆ Maxillary sinus below and anteriorly to it
    - ◆ Perpendicular plate of the palatine bone posteriorly to it

- Blood supply
  - ○ **Upper part:** Anterior and posterior ethmoidal branches of **ophthalmic** artery
  - ○ **Lower part:** Sphenopalatine branch of **maxillary artery** branch of external carotid artery and superior labial branch of the **facial artery.** Site of epistaxis
  - ○ Veins drain into cavernous sinus via facial and ophthalmic veins
- Nerve supply
  - ○ **Septum:** Long sphenopalatine nerve branch of maxillary branch of trigeminal nerve along with anterior ethmoidal nerve branch of nasociliary nerve from ophthalmic branch of trigeminal nerve
  - ○ **Upper lateral wall:** Short sphenopalatine nerve branch of maxillary branch of trigeminal nerve
  - ○ **Inferior lateral wall:** Superior dental nerve and the greater palatine nerve branches of maxillary branch of trigeminal nerve
  - ○ **Parasympathetic** supply to lacrimal glands comes from pterygopalatine ganglion

Muscle

4

Skeletal muscle

- **Anatomy:** Long tube-like multinucleated cells. Cell wall of muscle fibre cell is called sarcolemma. Each muscle fibre cell contains multiple myofibrils. Myofibrils are composed of adjacent blocks of actin and myosin known as sarcomere. Multiple invaginations of sarcolemma are called T-tubules, and they penetrate deep into cell
  - **Endomysium:** Connective tissue covering muscle cell fibres
  - **Perimysium:** Connective tissue covering fasciculus (group of muscle fibres)
  - **Epimysium:** Connective tissue covering muscle belly (group of fasciculi)
- **Thin myofilament:** Two molecules of actin and a molecule of **tropomyosin** in a helical arrangement. Each half-turn of this helix is bound by troponin. *Troponin is formed by three complexes:* troponin I, troponin T and troponin C
- **Thick myofilament:** Made up of *myosin.* Each myosin molecule has a tail and two head regions. Each head has an adenosine triphosphate (ATP)-binding site and an actin binding site
- Steps in muscle contraction
  - Nerve ending releases acetylcholine on depolarisation of nerve
  - Depolarisation of muscle cell happens and spreads in the sarcolemma to a deeper part of the cell through T-tubules
  - T-tubules cause release of Ca^{2+} from the sarcoplasmic reticulum (ryanodine receptors)

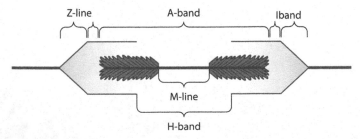

Figure 4.1 Skeletal muscle.

DOI: 10.1201/9781003390244-5

- Calcium binds to troponin C, which releases the tropomyosin from actin and allows binding of actin to the myosin-adenosine diphosphate (ADP)-Pi complex
- Binding of actin to myosin–ADP-Pi causes muscular contraction or power stroke, releasing an ADP-Pi molecule already attached to myosin
- At termination of muscle contraction, ATP binds to myosin, releasing actin and Ca^{2+}. Myosin retains the ADP-Pi. This is the same ADP-Pi that is released during the next cycle of the power stroke. Calcium goes back into sarcoplasmic reticulum and actin and myosin separate

	Type Ia	Type IIa	Type IIb
Colour	Red	Red	White
Myoglobin/Mitochondria	High	High	Low
Contraction speed	Slow	Medium	Fast
Metabolism	Fast oxidative	Slow oxidative	Fast glycolytic
Glycogen	Low	Moderate	High
Running	Marathon	Middle-distance	Sprint

Smooth muscle

- Involuntary muscle. Controlled by autonomic nervous system and hormones
- **Single-unit smooth muscle:** Coordinated contractions like in uterus and bowel
- **Multi-unit smooth muscle:** Iris, large arteries
- Smaller than striated muscle cells and arranged as sheets
- More actin and less myosin compared with striated muscle cells
- **Steps in muscle contraction**
  - Depolarisation of cell membrane causes opening of calcium channels in cell membrane (sodium channel opens in striated muscle)
  - Calcium binds to calmodulin in the cytoplasm as troponin is absent in smooth muscle cells
  - Calmodulin activates myosin light chain kinase (MLCK)
  - MLCK induces cross bridging of myosin and actin
  - Smooth muscle contracts more slowly than a striated muscle, but strength is greater due to the low ATPase activity of smooth muscle myosin

	Skeletal muscle	Cardiac muscle	Smooth muscle
Motor end plate	Yes	No	
T-tubule system	Well developed		Poorly developed
Mitochondria/Sarcoplasmic reticulum	Numerous		Few
Intercalated discs	Yes	No	Yes
Syncytium	No	Yes	
Blood supply	Abundant		Poor
Automaticity	No	Yes	Sometimes
Tetanic response	Yes	No	Yes
Response	All or none		Graded

Cardiac muscle

- Striated muscle similar to skeletal muscle but **branched**
- Individual cardiac muscle cells are tightly coupled to form a functional **syncytium**
- Not a true syncytium, as each cardiac muscle has a single nucleus and a separate sarcolemma
- Specialised end-to-end membrane junctions called **intercalated discs**
- Cardiac fibres offer a low resistance to propagation of action potentials due to intercalated discs
- All or nothing contractile response when myocardium is stimulated
- Cardiac muscles have more mitochondria than skeletal muscle
- Rapid contraction but no fatigue
- Specialised modified cardiomyocytes, known as pacemaker cells, set the rhythm of the heart contractions
- Steps in muscle contraction
  - Action potential at sarcolemma causes entry of Ca^{2+} to enter the cell from voltage and receptor-dependent channels (like smooth muscle cells)
  - Calcium is also released from sarcoplasmic reticulum
  - Calcium binds to troponin C and moves tropomyosin away from actin (like skeletal muscle cells)
  - Actin and myosin bind to each other causing contraction like skeletal muscle cells

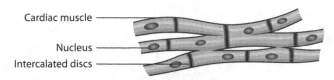

Figure 4.2   Cardiac muscle.

Neuromuscular junction

- **Neuromuscular junction (NMJ):** Consists of a muscle cell supplied by a motor neuron separated by a synaptic cleft
- **Synaptic cleft:** 20 nm wide
- 1–10 million acetylcholine receptors at each end plate
- Each vesicle contains 4–10,000 molecules of acetylcholine
- Each neuronal depolarisation releases roughly 200 vesicles
- Acetylcholine receptors can be nicotinic or muscarinic. Muscarinic receptors are G-protein-coupled receptors. Acetylcholine receptors at the NMJ are nicotinic receptors
- **Nicotinic acetylcholine receptor:** Transmembrane channel made up of five subunits including 2α, β, δ and ϵ. Subunits are arranged in a cylinder like structure with an ion channel in the centre
  - 2 Acetylcholines attach to two α subunits leading to the opening of the ion channel
- **Acetylcholine:** Synthesised from acetyl coenzyme A and choline. Enzyme choline acetyltransferase catalyses formation of acetylcholine. Stored in vesicles. Fusion of vesicles with nerve terminals is due to calcium
  - Acetylcholinesterase in synaptic cleft breaks down acetylcholine into acetate and choline
  - Acetylcholinesterase in plasma is known as pseudocholinesterase and causes breakdown of suxamethonium
- **Pre-junctional acetylcholine receptors:** Located in cell membrane of the nerve terminal. Activation of these receptors leads to release of further acetylcholine vesicles. Phase II block is characterised by impairment of pre-junctional acetylcholine release
- **Extra-junctional receptors:** Located just a bit distant from motor end plate. Significant in denervation injury, burns and muscle diseases
- **Botulinum:** Inhibition of acetylcholine release from nerve terminals

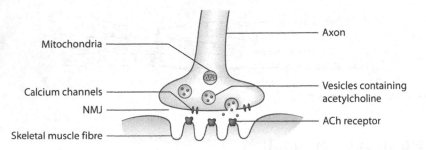

Figure 4.3 NMJ.

Muscle reflexes

- **Reflexes:** Involuntary, rapid, automatic responses to stimulus
- **Monosynaptic reflex:** Stretch reflex (knee jerk reflex) is an example. Tap the patellar tendon → stretching of quadriceps muscle → muscle spindle (sense organ) within the muscle lengthens → Ia/II afferent increases → spinal cord → Aα motor neuron → contraction of quadriceps muscle
  - ○ **Muscle spindle:** Provides background tone to muscles. *They respond to stretch of muscle*
    - ◆ Muscle spindles are present in belly of muscle
    - ◆ Afferent is Ia/II, which works like previously mentioned in the stretch reflex. Efferent is an Aγ nerve which causes contraction of muscle spindles and sets their sensitivities. Aγ is controlled by higher central nervous system (CNS) centres
    - ◆ Muscle spindles transduce muscle length
- **Inverse stretch reflex:** Relaxation (instead of contraction) of a muscle in response to a strong stretch. Too strong a tapping of the patellar tendon → muscle contraction (via complete stretch reflex) → sensing of tension by Golgi tendon organs → Ib afferent increases → spinal cord → Inhibition of efferent Aα motor neuron
  - ○ **Golgi tendon organs:** Prevents muscle damage
    - ◆ Golgi tendon organs as name suggests are near tendons of muscles
    - ◆ Afferent is Ib, which works as shown previously in inverse stretch reflex. They have no efferent supply
    - ◆ Golgi tendon organs transduce muscle force

- **Polysynaptic reflex:** Withdrawal reflex is an example. **Painful stimuli** → nociceptors → Aδ and C fibres → spinal cord → interneurons → Aα to both **flexor muscles of same limb** and **extensor muscles of contralateral limb**

  ○ Pain fibres ascend in contralateral spinothalamic tracts and synapse in the thalamus

- **Combined alphabetical and numerical nerve fibre classification**

Fibre types	Function
Aα	Motor neuron
Aβ	Touch, pressure
Aγ	Efferent to muscle spindle
Aδ	Sharp pain, temperature
B	Autonomic pre-ganglionic
C	Dull pain, temperature
Ia	Afferent from muscle spindle
Ib	Afferent from Golgi tendon organ
II	Afferent from muscle spindle
III	Pain, cold
IV	Pain, temperature

Gastrointestinal Tract

5

Nausea and vomiting

- **Nausea:** Uneasy sensation in the stomach that often accompanies the urge to vomit
- **Vomiting:** Vomiting is the forcible voluntary or involuntary emptying of stomach contents through the mouth
- **Vomiting centre:** Pool of loosely organised neurons in the medulla. Receives inputs from the following
  - **Limbic system:** Anxiety and extreme emotional state
  - **Chemoreceptor trigger zone (CTZ):** Lies in the floor of fourth ventricle in the area postrema within the dorsal surface of the medulla oblongata. Outside the blood–brain barrier (BBB)
    - Dopamine, D2
    - Serotonin, 5-HT_3
    - Acetylcholine, M_1
    - Histamine, H_1
    - Substance P, NK-1
    - Opioids, μ
  - **Cranial nerve VIII:** Vestibular labjyrinth. Motion sickness. Receptors involved
    - Acetylcholine, M_1
    - Histamine, H_1
  - **Cranial nerve X:** Baroreceptors (hypotension)
    - Gastrointestinal (GI) mucosa, 5-HT_3
  - **Cranial nerve IX:** Gag reflex
  - **Peripheral pain pathways**
- **Vomiting process**
  - **Pre-ejection phase:** Nausea
    - Sweating and tachycardia mediated by sympathetic nervous system
    - Salivation mediated by parasympathetic nervous system
    - Reverse peristalsis of the small intestine into stomach

DOI: 10.1201/9781003390244-6

- Retching phase: Deep inspiration followed by closure of glottis
  - Rhythmic contraction of the intercostal muscles, diaphragm and abdominal muscles against a closed glottis
- Ejection phase: Contraction of the pylorus, which pushes contents out of stomach
  - Relaxation of lower oesophageal sphincter (LOS)
- Risk factors for postoperative nausea and vomiting (PONV)
  - Patient factors: Female, children, non-smoker, history of PONV, history of motion sickness
  - Anaesthetic factors: Volatile agents, N_2O, opioids, high-dose neostigmine, hypotension
  - Surgical factors: Long-duration surgery, middle-ear surgery, eye surgery, laparoscopic surgery, gynaecology surgery
- Apfel score: 1 point each for female, history of PONV, non-smoker and postoperative opioids
  - 0 points = 9% risk, 1 point = 20% risk, 2 points = 39% risk, 3 points = 60% risk, 4 points = 78% risk

Swallowing and oesophagus

- Saliva: 500–1000 mL of saliva. 98% of saliva is water
  - pH is 8. Bicarbonate rich
  - α-Amylase: Breakdowns complex carbohydrates
  - Lingual lipase: Breakdowns dietary triglyceride
  - Haptocorrin: Binds vitamin B_{12} and protects it from the low pH of stomach
  - Lysozyme
  - Lactoferrin
  - Immunoglobin A
- Swallowing: The process that allows for a substance to pass from the mouth to the pharynx, and into the oesophagus, while shutting the epiglottis. Controlled by the medulla oblongata
  - Oral phase: The only voluntary phase of swallowing
    - Food touches the hard palate. Sensory information goes to medulla via glossopharyngeal nerve
  - Pharyngeal phase: Involuntary, controlled by medulla
    - Closure of the nasopharynx by the soft palate
    - Closure of laryngeal inlet and covering of inlet by epiglottis
    - 1–2 s of apnoea during swallowing

- Food bolus is propelled towards the oesophagus by successive contractions of the superior and middle pharyngeal constrictor muscles
- The inferior pharyngeal constrictor (cricopharyngeus/upper oesophageal sphincter [UOS]) muscles, which is normally closed, relaxes and allows the food to pass
  - Oesophageal phase: Involuntary
    - Once the food enters the oesophagus, UOS closes and the LOS opens
    - Food bolus is propelled along the oesophagus by peristalsis
- Oesophagus: Upper one-third of oesophagus is striated muscle and lower two-thirds is smooth muscle
  - UOS has a high resting pressure of up to 100 mm Hg
  - LOS has a pressure of 20–30 mm Hg
  - **Barrier pressure is difference between LOS pressure (20–30 mm Hg) and intragastric pressure (5–10 mm Hg). Barrier pressure of zero promoted reflux**
- Sphincters: A structure is usually made up of circular muscles. Sphincters can be
  - **Anatomical:** Different from the surrounding tissue, e.g., anal sphincter
  - **Functional: Similar like the surrounding tissue, e.g., LOS**
- LOS (cardiac sphincter): Functional sphincter at the junction of non-keratinised squamous epithelium of oesophagus and simple columnar epithelium of the stomach
  - Constricted at rest. Pressure of 20–30 mm Hg
  - LOS tone increased by cholinergic stimulation, histamine, gastrin and motilin
  - **LOS tone decreased by dopamine, oestrogen, cholecystokinin (CCK) and secretin**
- Anal sphincter: Anatomically an external ring of muscle at anorectal junction
  - **Internal anal sphincter:** Involuntary, will relax in response to stretching
  - **External anal sphincter:** Voluntary

Gastrointestinal digestion

- Gastric secretions: A total of 2 L per day
  - **Pepsinogen:** Produced by *chief cells*
    - Converted to pepsin by acidic environment of the stomach
    - Causes protein breakdown

- o Gastrin: Produced by G cells
  - ✦ Causes stimulation of parietal cells to produce hydrochloric acid (HCl)
  - ✦ Causes stimulation of chief cells to produce pepsinogen
  - ✦ Causes stimulation of gastric motility
- o HCl: Produced by *parietal cells*
  - ✦ *pH: 1–2. Active process by proton pump H+/K+-ATPase*
- o Mucus: Mucous cells secrete HCO_3^--rich mucus
  - ✦ Protects the gastric mucosa from the highly acidic contents of the stomach
- o Intrinsic factor (IF): Secreted by parietal cells
  - ✦ IF binds with vitamin B_{12} in duodenum
  - ✦ In the terminal ileum, IF receptors allow absorption of the IF–vitamin B_{12} complex
- • Phases of gastric regulation
  - o Cephalic phase: 30% of total gastric acid secreted per meal is produced in response to the smell and sight of food
    - ✦ Caused by vagal stimulation of gastric juices
  - o Gastric phase: 60% of total gastric acid secreted per meal is produced during gastric phase
    - ✦ Distension of stomach causes release of gastrin by G cells
  - o Intestinal phase: Chyme (food mixed with gastric juices) enters the duodenum
    - ✦ Secretin inhibits gastric secretion
    - ✦ CCK inhibits stomach emptying
    - ✦ Gastric inhibitory peptide (GIP) inhibits gastric motility
- • Nutrient reabsorption
  - o Carbohydrates: Salivary amylase in saliva breaks complex carbohydrates
    - ✦ Pancreatic amylase in duodenum also breaks complex carbohydrates
    - ✦ At brush border epithelium, sucrase, maltase and lactase break the carbohydrates into monosaccharides and absorbed
  - o Proteins: In stomach, pepsin cleaves proteins into smaller peptides
    - ✦ In duodenum, both trypsin and chymotrypsin released by pancreas, cleave polypeptides into dipeptides and tripeptides

- At brush border epithelium, peptidases break dipeptides into single amino acids and absorbed
  - **Lipids:** In duodenum, bile acids secreted by liver emulsify big lipid droplets into smaller droplets
    - Pancreatic lipase hydrolyses triglyceride molecules into free fatty acids (FFAs) and glycerides
    - FFAs and glycerides combine with bile salts forming micelles and absorbed
    - Dietary fat and water are absorbed throughout the small intestine
  - Iron is absorbed in the duodenum
  - **Vitamin B_{12} and bile salts are absorbed in the terminal ileum**
- **Pancreas:** 1.5 L of pancreatic juice is produced per day
  - Endocrine function: 1–2% of the pancreatic mass. Islets of Langerhans
    - α **cells:** Glucagon
    - β **cells:** Insulin
    - δ **cells:** Somatostatin
  - **Exocrine functions: Acinar cells**
    - **Trypsinogen and chymotrypsinogen:** First enterokinase, a duodenal enzyme, cleaves them into trypsin and chymotrypsin. Trypsin then further cleaves both trypsinogen and chymotrypsinogen
    - Pancreatic amylase
    - Pancreatic lipase
- **Bile:** 1000 mL of bile is produced by liver per day. Concentrated to 200 mL by gallbladder
  - **Constituents:** Bile salts, bile pigments, water, electrolytes, cholesterol and phospholipids
  - **Bile pigments:** In spleen, red blood cell (RBC) $\rightarrow$ haemoglobin $\rightarrow$ haem (Fe^{2+} and porphyrin ring) and globin $\rightarrow$ porphyrin $\rightarrow$ biliverdin $\rightarrow$ bilirubin. This bilirubin is transported to liver bound to albumin
    - Bilirubin $\rightarrow$ bile pigments, which undergo enterohepatic circulation
  - **Bile acids: Produced by oxidation of cholesterol**
    - Na^+ and K^+ salts of bile acids are called bile salts
    - Emulsification of dietary lipids
    - Fat-soluble vitamins A, D, E and K are absorbed by this micelle forming bile salts
    - Bile salts are reabsorbed at the terminal ileum

Hormone	Produced by	Released due to	Actions
Gastrin	G cells in stomach	- Cephalic phase (vagus nerve) - Stomach distension - Partially digested proteins	- ↑ Pepsinogen - ↑ Acid - ↑ Gastric motility - ↑ Lower oesophageal sphincter tone
Secretin	S cells of duodenum	- Acidic chyme in small intestine	- ↑ Pancreatic enzymes release - ↑ Release of bile from gallbladder - ↑ Enhances action of CCK
CCK	I cells of duodenum	- Amino acids and fatty acids in small intestine	- ↑ Pancreatic enzymes release - ↑ Release of bile from gallbladder - ↑ Enhances action of secretin - ↑ Feeling of satiety - ↓ Gastric emptying
GIP	K cells of duodenum	- Fatty acids in small intestine	- ↓ Gastric emptying - ↓ Gastric juices - ↑ Insulin release

- **Acid secretion:** Increased by food, stress, alcohol, caffeine, **histamine** and **gastrin**
  - Decreased by fatty acids, glucose and amino acids in small intestine, vagotomy, CCK, GIP and secretin
- **Gastric emptying:** Increased by metoclopramide and neostigmine
  - Decreased by food, alcohol, stress, old age
- **Small intestinal motility:** Both the nervous and endocrine system
  - **The enteric nervous system:** Operates semi-autonomously, with inputs from sympathetic and parasympathetic nervous system. Neurons converge on two ganglia
    - **Meissner's plexus:** Submucosal in location
    - **Auerbach's plexus:** Myenteric location
  - **The endocrine system**
    - CCK
    - Gastrin

- Motilin: Hormone released from duodenum every 90 min during fasting that stimulates the gastric and intestinal motility
- **Vasoactive intestinal peptide (VIP):** Increases secretion of water and electrolytes in the small intestine. Stimulates intestinal motility

Splanchnic blood supply

- Aorta: Has three branches through which it supplies the gut
- Coeliac artery: T12 level. Small 1.25-cm vessel
  - Common hepatic artery
  - Left gastric artery
  - **Splenic artery**
- Superior mesenteric artery: L1 level
  - Pancreaticoduodenal artery
  - Intestinal artery
  - Ileocolic artery
  - Right colic artery
  - **Middle colic artery**
- Inferior mesenteric artery: L3 level
  - Left colic artery
  - Sigmoid artery
  - **Superior rectal artery**
- **Venous structures**
  - Oesophagus is drained by branches of the azygous veins and the inferior thyroid vein
  - Mesenteric circulation drains via the superior and inferior mesenteric vein. These two vessels are joined by the splenic vein to form the portal vein. Portal vein then splits to form the right and left branches in the liver. From the portal vein, blood drains via the hepatic vein into the inferior vena cava (IVC)
  - **Lower third of the rectum and anus drain into the middle rectal vein, which drains directly into the IVC**
- **Splanchnic nerves: Sympathetic nerves supplying GI tract (GIT)**
  - **Greater splanchnic nerve: T5–T9**
  - **Lesser splanchnic nerve: T10–T11**
  - **Least splanchnic nerve: T12**
- **Vagus nerve:** Parasympathetic nerve supplying GIT

- Splanchnic blood flow (SBF) is normally 30 mL/min/100 g ~ 25–30% of cardiac output
- Oxygen extraction is low ~10%
- Regulation of SBF
  - Intrinsic control
    1. *Metabolic:* H^+, K^+, adenosine and CO_2
    2. Myogenic
  - Extrinsic control
    1. *Neurogenic:* Autonomic nervous system containing the sympathetic nervous system and parasympathetic nervous system
    2. *Humoral control:* Vasodilators like gastrin, secretin, CCK, VIP, substance P, prostaglandins, nitric oxide (NO), dopamine and vasoconstrictors like vasopressin, angiotensin II, peptide YY, neuropeptide YY
- Normal intra-abdominal pressure (IAP) is 5–7 mm Hg
- Intra-abdominal hypertension is IAP >12 mm Hg
- Abdominal compartment syndrome is IAP >20 mm Hg

Liver

- **Liver anatomy:** Liver weighs around 1500–2000 g. **Normal portal venous pressure: 5–10 mm Hg**
  - **Couinaud** divided liver into eight independent functional segments with each segment having its own hepatic arterial branch, portal branch and a bile duct with separate hepatic venous outflow
    - **Caudate lobe:** Segment I
    - **Left lobe:** Segments II–IV
    - **Right lobe:** Segments V–VIII
  - Histological unit: *Lobule.* Hexagonal in shape with *hepatic vein at centre* and portal triads at the periphery
    - **Portal triad:** Hepatic artery, portal vein and bile duct
    - Sinusoids take blood from portal triad to the central vein and contain Kupffer cells (reticuloendothelial cells)
  - Functional unit: Acinus. Diamond shaped. **Area between two central veins that is formed by triangular portions of adjacent lobules**
    - Zone 1: Close to portal triad. Mitochondria rich. Oxidative metabolism and glycogen synthesis
    - Zone 2: Between areas 1 and 3

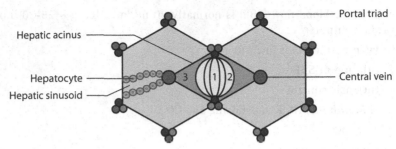

Figure 5.1 Hepatic acinus.

- ● Zone 3: Close to central vein. Prone to ischaemia. Smooth endoplasmic reticulum rich. Cytochrome P450 for drug and toxin biotransformation
- **Blood supply of liver:** 1.5 L/min. 25% of cardiac output
  - ○ *Hepatic portal vein:* 75% of liver's blood supply, 50% of oxygen requirements
  - ○ *Hepatic artery:* 25% of liver's blood supply, 50% of oxygen requirements
- **Autoregulation of hepatic blood flow:** Blood flow through hepatic artery is autoregulated to maintain a constant flow mean arterial pressure (MAP) between 60 and 160 mm Hg
  - ○ *Intrinsic control*
    1. **Metabolic:** NO causes vasodilation
    2. **Myogenic:** Direct contractile response of the hepatic arterial smooth muscle to stretch and vice versa
    3. **Hepatic arterial buffer response:** Hepatic artery dilates or constricts compared with changes in blood flow in portal vein to maintain constant blood flow
  - ○ *Extrinsic control*
    1. **Neurogenic:** Autonomic nervous system containing the sympathetic nervous system and parasympathetic nervous system
    2. **Surgical handling:** Reduces hepatic blood flow
- **Functions of liver**
  1. **Biotransformation:** Metabolism of drugs and toxins
  2. **Synthetic function**
     - ● Albumin and all globulins except gamma globulins
     - ● C-reactive protein
     - ● Clotting factors except factor VIII

- Antithrombin III
- Immunoglobins

3. **Storage:** Glycogen
   - Copper
   - Iron as ferritin
   - Vitamins A, D, E and K and B_{12}

4. **Metabolism**
   - **Carbohydrates:** Gluconeogenesis, glycogenolysis, glycogenesis
   - **Urea:** Proteins are synthesis, transamination and deaminated and waste products are excreted as urea
   - **Ketone bodies:** Lipolysis to produce acetoacetate and β-hydroxybutyrate
   - **Lipids:** Cholesterol synthesis, high-density lipoprotein (HDL) and low-density lipoprotein (LDL) metabolism
   - **Vitamins:** Activates vitamin D (25-hydroxylation)

5. **Exocrine:** Bile needed for emulsification of dietary lipids
   - Bile is needed for absorption of fat-soluble vitamins A, D, E and K

6. **Endocrine:** Secretes hormones angiotensinogen, thrombopoietin and insulin-like growth factor-1 (IGF-1)

7. **Capacitance:** Liver can hold up to 15% of the circulating volume as blood reservoir

- **Liver function tests (LFTs)**
  - **Hepatic LFTs:** Alanine transaminase (ALT) and aspartate transaminase (AST) released in blood following hepatocellular damage
    - AST found in heart and skeletal muscle and less specific
    - **Alcohol liver disease:** AST:ALT ratio >2:1. Typically ALT <300 U/L
    - A raised ALT of >1000 U/L is seen in ischaemic hepatitis, drug-induced liver injury (paracetamol, statins, non-steroidal anti-inflammatory drugs [NSAIDs], methotrexate), acute viral hepatitis, autoimmune hepatitis
  - **Cholestatic LFTs:** Predominant increase in alkaline phosphatase ± a rise in bilirubin
    - Gamma-glutamyl transferase (GGT) is more liver specific as ALP is produced by both bones and liver
    - **Extrahepatic biliary obstruction:** Gallstones, pancreatic head cancer
    - **Intrahepatic biliary obstruction:** Primary biliary cholangitis (PBC), primary sclerosing cholangitis (PSC), medications like steroids, oral contraceptives (OCPs), flucloxacillin, co-amoxiclav

○ Synthetic functions

  ♦ **Albumin:** Reduced in chronic liver disease. May be lost in renal and GI losses, hence, not specific

  ♦ **International normalised ratio (INR):** All clotting factors except factor VIII are synthesised by the liver; hence, it is used to indirectly assess liver function

Jaundice

Jaundice: Yellowing of skin, sclera and mucous membranes due to accumulation of bilirubin in blood.

- **Normal bilirubin:** 17 μmol/L
- **Clinically detectable:** 34–51 μmol/L (two to three times the normal values)

Bilirubin metabolism

- Haemoglobin broken into haem and globin. Haem is turned into biliverdin, which is converted into bilirubin
- Unconjugated bilirubin binds to albumin in the circulation and is transported to liver
- Bilirubin conjugated with glucuronic acid and this water-soluble bilirubin diglucuronide is excreted via bile canaliculi into the duodenum
- In the intestine, 95% of bilirubin is reabsorbed and undergoes enterohepatic circulation
- Bilirubin converted to stercobilinogen by colonic bacteria, which is excreted in faeces as stercobilin or urine as urobilinogen

Causes of jaundice

- **Pre-hepatic (unconjugated):**
  ○ Haemolytic anaemia
  ○ Physiological jaundice of newborns
  ○ Gilbert's disease (decreased activity of uridine diphosphate [UDP] glucuronosyltransferase)
  ○ Crigler–Najjar syndrome (deficiency of UDP glucuronosyltransferase)
- **Hepatic (unconjugated or conjugated)**
  ○ Liver failure (unconjugated)
  ○ Dubin–Johnson syndrome (lesions of gene *MRP2* involved in canalicular transport) (conjugated)
  ○ Rotor syndrome (defective protein OATP1B1 and OATP1B3 involved in hepatic storage of bilirubin) (conjugated)
  ○ Drugs: OCPs, anabolic steroids, haloperidol

- Post-hepatic (conjugated)
  - Gallstones
  - Pancreatic carcinoma
  - PBC
  - PSC

Spleen

- Size of an adult fist, 11–12 cm in craniocaudal length and weighs 150 g
- Lies along the 9th, 10th and 11th ribs on left side
- **Arterial supply:** Splenic artery, which is a branch of the coeliac trunk
- **Venous drainage:** Splenic vein drains it and joins superior mesenteric vein to form the portal vein
- **Gastrosplenic ligament:** Short gastric and the gastroepiploic vessels along with sympathetic nerves from the coeliac plexus
- **Lienorenal ligament:** Splenic vessels
- **White pulp:** Lymphatic nodules around an arteriole
- **Red pulp:** RBCs, macrophages and lymphocytes

Functions
- **Red cell storage:** Around 8%
- **Lymphopoiesis:** Lymphocytes to plasma cells
- **Phagocytosis:** Removes ageing red cells, platelets
- **Haematopoiesis:** During fetal life

Effects of splenectomy
- **RBC:** Howell–Jolly bodies, erythroblasts
- **WBC:** Leucocytosis
- **Platelet:** Thrombocytosis, increased adhesiveness
- Immunological defects
  - $\downarrow$ Serum IgM levels
  - $\downarrow$ Level of phagocyte-promoting peptide
  - **Response to particulate antigens**

Kidney

- **Kidney facts:** Each kidney has 1.2 million nephrons
  - 15% of nephrons are juxtamedullary, which means that loops of Henle and collecting ducts project down into the medulla

- ○ Glomerular filtration rate (GFR): *125 mL/min* or 180 L/day
- ○ Renal blood flow (RBF) = 1.2 L/min
- ○ Renal plasma flow (RPF)= 600 mL/min
- ○ Filtration fraction = GFR/RPF = 0.2
- ○ 20% of cardiac output
- ○ *Weigh 300 g total. Hence highest blood flow per gram of tissue*
- ○ **Blood flow:** Renal cortex is 500 mL/min/100 g. Renal medulla is 100 mL/min/100 g
- ○ Transport maximum (T_{max}) for glucose is 11 mmol/L
- ○ *Molecular weight >70 kDa: Not filtered, hence, no albumin*
- ○ Urine specific gravity: 1010–1035
- ○ Urine osmolality of 700 = specific gravity of 1020
- **Nephron:** Glomerulus, proximal convoluted tubule (PCT), loop of Henle, distal convoluted tubule (DCT) and collecting duct
  - ○ **Glomerulus:** GFR measured using **inulin ideally** and creatinine clearance clinically
    - ◆ Fick principle used or calculated using Cockcroft–Gault equation
    - ◆ **Clearance (GFR) = Urine concentration of inulin or creatinine × Urine flow/Plasma concentration**
    - ◆ **Decreased by:** Vasopressin, noradrenaline, prostaglandins, leukotrienes, histamine
    - ◆ **Increased by:** Dilatation of afferent arteriole and constriction of efferent arteriole, dopamine, atrial natriuretic peptide (ANP)
  - ○ **PCT:** Reabsorbs 60% of the ultrafiltrate and calcium
    - ◆ 65% of filtered sodium, water and chloride
    - ◆ 55% of filtered potassium
    - ◆ *100% of filtered glucose and amino acids*
    - ◆ 85% of filtered bicarbonate
    - ◆ 90% of filtered phosphate
    - ◆ Uric acid is also filtered
    - ◆ Na^+/amino acid symporters help reabsorption of sodium and amino acids in blood. This is at the apical membrane towards the lumen of PCT
    - ◆ Sodium-glucose linked transporters (SGLTs) help reabsorption of sodium and glucose in blood. This is at the apical membrane
    - ◆ Na^+/K^+-ATPase functions to bring in 2 K^+ and pump out 3 Na^+ towards blood vessels at the basolateral membrane

- Na$^+$/H$^+$ antiporter: Sodium reabsorption is active with a counter transport of H$^+$ secretion into lumen of PCT. This is at the apical membrane
- H$^+$ secretion into lumen allows reabsorption of bicarbonate via the use of the enzyme carbonic anhydrase
- Therefore, for every one molecule of H$^+$ secreted, one molecule of bicarbonate and Na$^+$ is reabsorbed into the bloodstream
- Water is reabsorbed along with sodium to make sure that osmolality is maintained
- Potassium, urea and chloride are reabsorbed by passive diffusion
- *Urine before it enters the loop of Henle has an osmolality of about 300 mOsmol/L*
- *At the distal end of the PCT, tubular concentration of sodium and plasma concentration of sodium are equal*
  - Loop of Henle: Counter current multiplier magic happens here
    - *Gradient is 1400 mOsmol/kg H$_2$O* at the tip of the loop
    - Urine osmolality leaving the loop of Henle is 100 mOsmol/kg H$_2$O
    - Thin descending limb of Henle is permeable to water, so only water is reabsorbed
    - Thick and thin ascending limbs of Henle are impermeable to water
    - At ascending loop of Henle, frusemide-sensitive Na$^+$/K$^+$/Cl$^-$ cotransport helps to reabsorb these ions from lumen into blood
  - DCT: Has a thiazide-sensitive Na$^+$-Cl$^-$ cotransporter, which helps absorb sodium from the lumen side
    - Calcium regulation is done by reabsorbing Ca^{2+} in response to parathyroid hormone
  - The collecting duct: Aldosterone increases reabsorption of sodium by excreting hydrogen and potassium ions
    - Antidiuretic hormone (ADH) increases water reabsorption
- Autoregulation of RBF: Constant RBF with a MAP between 70 and 180 mm Hg
  - *Intrinsic control*
    1. Metabolic: NO and renal prostaglandins cause vasodilation
    2. Myogenic: Direct contractile response of the afferent arteriolar smooth muscle to stretch
    3. Tubuloglomerular feedback: Macula densa in the distal tubular epithelium detects the sodium ion within the tubule and causes stimulation of vascular smooth muscle in the afferent arteriole

- ○ *Extrinsic control*
  1. **Neurogenic:** Autonomic nervous system containing the sympathetic nervous system and parasympathetic nervous system
  2. **Hormonal:** Angiotensin II vasoconstricts the efferent arteriole more than the afferent arteriole, hence, it maintains GFR
- **RBF calculation:** Calculated using the Fick principle, which says that blood flow to an organ is equal to the uptake/excretion of a substance by an organ per unit time divided by the difference of arteriovenous concentration
  - ○ Clearance of PAH = Urine [PAH] × Urine flow/Renal plasma flow
  - ○ RBF = RPF/1 – Hct

    where PAH is para-aminohippurate, RPF is renal plasma flow and Hct is haematocrit.
- **Hormones produced by kidney**
  - ○ Renin
  - ○ Erythropoietin
  - ○ Vitamin D (1-hydroxylation)
- **Glomerular filtration pressures**
  - ○ **Plasma oncotic pressure:** 25–30 mm Hg, Bowman's capsule oncotic pressure is zero
  - ○ **Afferent and efferent arteriolar pressure:** 50 mm Hg
  - ○ **Hydrostatic pressure in Bowman's capsule:** 10–15 mm Hg
  - ○ **Renal venous pressure:** <5 mm Hg

#Chronic kidney disease causes normochromic, normocytic anaemia.

Endocrine

6

Pituitary

- Pea sized, 0.5 g
- Sits at the base of the brain in the sella turcica
- Anterior pituitary (adenohypophysis) (chromophil cells)
  - Develops from Rathke's pouch (oral ectoderm in roof of developing mouth)
  - Adrenocorticotropic (ACTH), thyroid-stimulating hormone (TSH), follicle-stimulating hormone (FSH), luteinising hormone (LH), prolactin, growth hormone (GH)
- Posterior pituitary (neurohypophysis)
  - Develops from neural ectoderm from floor of hypothalamus
  - Neurons from the supraoptic and paraventricular nucleus of the hypothalamus synthesize the hormones and then travel down the nerve axon connecting the posterior pituitary
  - Secretes ADH (*nonapeptide,* supraoptic) and oxytocin (nonapeptide, paraventricular)
- Arterial supply
  - Superior and inferior hypophyseal arteries from internal carotid artery
- Portal circulation
  - The pooling of blood from one capillary bed to another without first going through the heart
  - The hypophyseal portal system links the hypothalamus and the anterior pituitary
  - Similar system is hepatic portal circulation
- Pituitary adenomas
  - Microadenomas <1 cm and macroadenomas >1 cm
- Antidiuretic hormone (ADH)
  - Morphine, barbiturates, and nicotine cause ADH secretion
  - Alcohol inhibits ADH secretion
  - Released in response to increase in serum osmolality sensed by hypothalamic osmoreceptors
  - Hypovolemia via baroreceptors also stimulates ADH secretion

In central polyuria, use I/V DDAVP to treat it.

DOI: 10.1201/9781003390244-7

Thyroid

- **Butterfly-shaped gland,** Level C5-C7/T1
  - Two lobes joined by an isthmus just below the level of cricoid cartilage overlying 2nd to 4th tracheal rings
  - Lateral lobes extend from middle of thyroid cartilage until the 4th to 6th tracheal rings
- *Arterial supply* via
  - Superior thyroid artery (external carotid artery)
  - Inferior thyroid artery (thyrocervical trunk)
  - Thyroid ima, 10% (brachiocephalic trunk)
- *Venous drainage* via
  - Superior thyroid veins (internal jugular vein)
  - Middle thyroid veins (internal jugular vein)
  - Inferior thyroid veins (left brachiocephalic vein)
- A dense capillary plexus is present deep to the true capsule. To avoid haemorrhage during surgery, the thyroid is removed along with the capsule. In the prostate the venous plexus lies between two capsules; therefore, during prostatectomy, both capsules are left behind
- Principal hormones – Thyroxine (T4), Triiodothyronine (T3) and calcitonin
  - Thyroid gland takes in iodide ion by active transport, and peroxidase converts this iodide ion to atomic Iodine. Atomic iodine is added to tyrosine forming mono- or diiodo tyrosine. These iodinated tyrosine residues couple up to form T4 or T3
  - **T3 and T4 remain attached to thyroglobulin and are stored as colloid**
  - Up to 80% of the T4 is converted to T3 by peripheral organs such as liver, kidney and spleen
  - T3 is 10 times more active than T4
  - Only 0.02% of T4 and 0.3% of T3 is biologically active
  - The rest is bound to plasma proteins like thyroid-binding globulin, transthyretin and albumin
  - T3 is responsible for 80% of metabolic activity
  - Half-life of T4 is 7 days and T3 is 1 day
- Functions of thyroid hormones
  - **Metabolic:** Increases basal metabolic rate (BMR), sensitivity to catecholamines, breakdown of proteins and increased turnover of calcium from bone
  - **Growth:** Permissive effect on growth hormone
  - **Nervous system:** Normal development

- **Regulation:** Hypothalamus releases thyroid-releasing hormone (TRH), which causes release of TSH from the anterior pituitary. TSH causes release of T4/T3, which has a negative feedback effect on the hypothalamus and pituitary
- **Hyperthyroidism:** Tachycardia, atrial fibrillation, hypertension, high output cardiac failure, tremors, restlessness, exophthalmos, lid lag, ophthalmoplegia, weight loss, oligo/amenorrhoea, proximal muscle wasting
- **Hypothyroid:** Bradycardia, peripheral oedema, ischaemic heart disease, hypertension, slow reflexes, ataxia, weight gain, constipation, infertility, proximal myopathy

Adrenals

- Suprarenal glands at level of T12 vertebra
- Divided into two parts
  - Adrenal cortex: Outer part of gland. Produces corticosteroid hormones
    - Zona glomerulosa: Outermost. Mineralocorticoids (aldosterone)
    - Zona fasciculata: Middle part. Glucocorticoids (cortisol)
    - Zona reticularis: Innermost. Androgens (dehydroepiandrosterone)

#Cushing syndrome: Hypertension, hypernatremia, hypokalaemia, and hyperglycaemia. Glucose intolerance not seen much in Conn's syndrome.

  - Adrenal medulla: Inner part of the gland. Chromaffin cells
    - 20% Noradrenaline and 80% adrenaline
- **Glucocorticoids:** Normal output of 25 mg cortisol daily
  - Effects
    - ↑ Glycogen, protein and fat catabolism → ↑ glucose
    - Hepatic gluconeogenesis → ↑ glucose
    - Increased sensitivity of cardiovascular system to catecholamines
    - Suppresses immune system
    - Anti-inflammatory system
  - Regulation
    - Corticotropin-releasing hormone (CRH) and ACTH are released by the hypothalamus and pituitary, respectively. CRH increases ACTH and ACTH increases cortisol. Both are inhibited negatively by cortisol
- Prednisolone ≥5 mg/day in adults or equivalent dose can cause suppression of the hypothalamic-pituitary-adrenal axis. These patients require intraoperative corticosteroids

- **Aldosterone:** Acts on mineralocorticoid receptor (MR) and increases the reabsorption of sodium and excretion of potassium from principal cells of the distal convoluted tubule (DCT) of the kidney
  - Both sodium and water are reabsorbed; hence, urinary osmolality doesn't change
  - Regulation
    - **Plasma ACTH:** Increases aldosterone
    - **Renin-angiotensin-aldosterone (RAA) system:** ↓ circulatory volume causes ↓ renal afferent arteriolar pressure leading to ↑ renin secretion from juxtaglomerular cells. Renin cleaves angiotensinogen (liver) into angiotensin I. Angiotensin I is converted into angiotensin II by angiotensin-converting enzyme (ACE) produced by the lungs. **Angiotensin II increases aldosterone**
    - **Fall in plasma sodium concentration:** ↓ Na⁺ detected by macula densa in DCT, causing secretion of aldosterone
- **Catecholamines:** Tyrosine hydroxylase is the rate-limiting step of converting tyrosine to DOPA

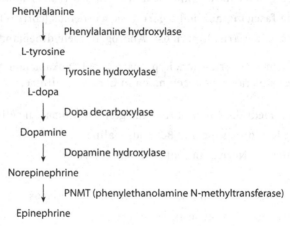

Figure 6.1   Catecholamines.

Metabolism

7

Acid-base balance

- **Acid:** Acid is a molecule that is a proton donor
- **Base:** Acid is a molecule that is a proton acceptor or hydroxide (OH^-) donor
- **pH:** Negative logarithm to base 10 of hydrogen ion concentration
  - $pH = -\log_{10}[H^+]$
  - At pH of 7.4, $[H^+]$ = 40 nmol/L
- **pKa:** pH of an acid at which it is 50% dissociated or in equilibrium with its base
- **Standard bicarbonate:** Concentration of bicarbonate when arterial $PaCO_2$ has been corrected to 5.3 kPa, haemoglobin being fully saturated and the body temperature at 37°C
- **Base excess (deficit):** The amount of acid or base that will restore 1 L of blood to normal pH at a $PaCO_2$ of 5.3 kPa and at body temperature
- Solubility factor for carbon dioxide in plasma = 0.225 mmol/L/kPa
- **Henderson–Hasselbach equation:** pH = pKa + log [conjugate base/acid] = pKa + log [A⁻]/[HA]
- **Blood buffers**
  - **Bicarbonate/carbonic acid:** Important extracellular and blood buffer system
    - pKa is 6.1
    - More efficient in buffering acids
  - **Haemoglobin:** Important blood buffer system
    - pKa is 6.8
    - **Imidazole group of histidine of haemoglobin accepts hydrogen ions**
    - Six times the buffering capacity of plasma proteins
  - **Phosphate:** Small role in extracellular fluid (ECF) but important intracellular buffer
    - pKa is 6.8
  - **Proteins:** Extracellular and blood buffer system
    - pKa is 2 for carboxyl group and 9 for amino group

DOI: 10.1201/9781003390244-8

- Urinary buffering
  - **Bicarbonate/carbonic acid:** Happens in proximal convolutional tubule (PCT)
  - **Phosphate ($HPO_4^-/H_2PO_4^-$):** Some in PCT but most in distal convolutional tubule (DCT)
  - **Ammonia (NH_3/NH_4^-):** PCT and DCT
  - Buffering by bicarbonate results in bicarbonate reabsorption, whereas buffering with phosphate and ammonia results in bicarbonate regeneration
- **Bone buffering**
  - Release of calcium carbonate from bone is the most important buffering mechanism involved in chronic metabolic acidosis

In acute metabolic acidosis, respiratory function is the vital component of bicarbonate/carbonic acid buffer system.

Anion gap

- **Anion gap:** Difference between measured cations and measured anions in serum
- Difference can be due to presence of unmeasured anions such as lactate, ketones
- AG = $\{[Na^+] + [K^+]\} - \{[Cl^-] + [HCO_3^-]\}$
- Normal range = 10–20 mmol/L
- **High anion gap metabolic acidosis [MUDPILES]**
  - Methanol
  - Uraemia
  - Diabetic ketoacidosis
  - Propylene glycol
  - Iron/Isoniazid
  - Lactic acidosis
  - Ethylene glycol
  - Salicylates
- **Normal anion gap metabolic acidosis [CAGE]**
  - Chloride excess
  - Acetazolamide/Addison's
  - Gastrointestinal (GI) causes – diarrhoea/vomiting
  - Extrarenal tubular acidosis
  - Urinary anion gap to differentiate between a GI and renal cause of a normal anion gap acidosis. Urinary anion gap = $Na^+ + K^+ - Cl^-$. Renal

causes have increased urinary HCO_3^- excretion, increasing urinary anion gap; whereas GI causes have increased $NH4^+$ excretion, decreasing urinary anion gap

- **Lactic acid:** Normally produced in the body at 20 mmol/kg/day as a by-product of metabolism. It is metabolised by the liver and kidney. Excess lactates can cause acidosis
- **Hyperlactatemia:** Lactate levels between 2 and 4 mmol/L. Severe levels are >4 mmol/L
- **Lactate acidosis:** Metabolic acidosis associated with raised plasma lactate concentration (>2 mmol/L)
  - **Type A:** Due to tissue hypoxia (all types of shocks), which leads to anaerobic glycolysis
  - **Type B:** Non-hypoxic causes, e.g., liver disease, malignancy, medications (metformin, salbutamol, epinephrine), total parenteral nutrition (TPN), diabetic ketoacidosis (DKA), ethanol intoxication, thiamine deficiency

Fluid compartments

- **Total body water (TBW):** 60% of body weight in men and 50% in women
  - Females are proportionately fatter than men
  - Neonates have a lower percentage of body fat and more water proportion
- **Intracellular fluid (ICF):** Two-thirds of total body weight. 40% of body weight in men
- **ECF:** One-third of total body weight. 20% of body weight in men
  - ECF = plasma volume (5%) + interstitial fluid (15%)
- **Transcellular fluid:** Secreted fluid separated from plasma by a layer of epithelium, e.g., cerebrospinal fluid (CSF), bile, intraocular fluids. Approximately 1 L
- **Composition of major body fluids**

	Plasma (mmol/L)	Intracellular fluid (mmol/L)
Na^+	145	10
Cl^+	110	3
K^+	4	155
Ca^+	3	1
Mg^+	1	40
HCO_3^-	26	7
Proteins	10	45

- Measurement of fluid compartments

Compartment	Indicator
Total body water (TBW)	• For example, **deuterium**, antipyrine • Distributed freely across all compartments
Extracellular fluid (ECF)	• For example, **inulin,** mannitol, sucrose • Does not enter the cell
Intracellular fluid	TBW – ECF
Plasma	• For example, Evan's blue, **radioiodinated serum albumin (RISA)** • Remains in plasma only
Red cell volume	• For example, ^{51}Cr-labelled red cells
Interstitial fluid	• ECF – Plasma volume

- Active transport: Movement against a concentration gradient at expenditure of energy
  - Saturable process and increases as body temperature increases
  - Movement of sodium out of a cell, iodide trapping, acid secretion by gastric cells

Fluid	Osmolarities (mOsm/L)
0.9% Saline	310
Hartmann's solution	278
5% Dextrose	280
10% Dextrose	560
0.18% Saline/4% Glucose	255
4.5% Albumin	330
20% Albumin	135
10% Mannitol	550
8.4% $NaHCO_3$	2000

Carbohydrate metabolism

- *Glycolysis*: Breakdown of glucose to produce energy
  - **Embden–Meyerhof–Parnas (EMP) pathway/glycolysis:** Glucose (C6) metabolised into two molecules of pyruvates (C3) along with net production of 2 ATPs + 2 NADH
    - Glucose → G-6P → F-6P → F-1,6 diphosphate →→→ 2 molecules of pyruvate

- Under aerobic conditions, pyruvate (C3) is oxidised to acetyl CoA (C2) with production of one more NADH per molecule oxidised, with a total 4 NADH + 2 ATPs at the end of glucose to acetyl CoA

- Under anaerobic conditions, pyruvate is converted to lactate, where 1 NADH is consumed per molecule metabolised; hence, the 2 NADH produced before from glucose to pyruvate are consumed and just 2 ATPs are the net benefit. **Catalysed by lactate dehydrogenase (LDH). LDH is found in muscle, heart and liver**

  - **Krebs cycle/citric acid cycle/tricarboxylic acid:** Acetyl CoA (C2) enters the cycle by reacting with oxaloacetate (C4) to form citrate (C6)

    - Acetyl CoA (C4) + oxaloacetate (C2) → citrate (C6) → α-ketoglutarate (C5) → succinate (C4) → oxaloacetate (C4)

    - 3 NADH, 1 $FADH_2$ and 1 ATP are produced per molecule, hence, a total of 6 NADH, 2 $FADH_2$ and 2 ATPs are produced

    - Therefore, under aerobic conditions 10 NADH, 2 $FADH_2$ and 4 ATPs overall are produced

  - **Oxidative phosphorylation:** The electron transport chain uses the NADH and $FADH_2$ to make ATPs. NADH produces 3 ATPs and $FADH_2$ produces 2 ATPs

    - 10 NADH = 10×3 = 30, 2 $FADH_2$ = 2×2 = 4. A total of 34 ATPs are produced and net gain adding 4 ATPs = 34 + 4 =38 ATPs

- *Glycogenolysis*: Breakdown of glycogen stores to produce glucose

  - **Skeletal muscle:** Glucose for muscular contraction

  - **Liver:** Glucose for glycolysis

- *Gluconeogenesis*: **Production of glucose from lactate and amino acids**

  - **Cori cycle:** Lactate produced in muscle is converted to glucose in liver and kidney (minor)

Cholesterol metabolism

- Used for synthesis of both steroid and bile acids
- Constituent of lipoprotein matrix of cell membrane with *no intrinsic hormonal activity* of its own
- Present in blood mainly as non-ester lipoprotein complex

Respiratory quotient

- Carbohydrate: 1
- Protein: 0.8
- Fats: 0.7

Starvation

- *Starvation:* Absent or inadequate nutrition resulting in the body to use its own endogenous stores. Can result in death in 60 days
- Body response to starvation
  - Behavioural: Reduction in spontaneous physical activity
  - Metabolic: Glycogenolysis, gluconeogenesis and ketogenesis
- Well-fed state: Brain accounts for 70–80% of glucose utilised at rest
  - Resting muscles utilize free fatty acids
- First 24 hours of fasting
  - Blood glucose to brain is a priority
  - Liver has 50–120 g of glycogen and muscle has 350–400 g of glycogen
  - *Glycogen reserves are over in 24–48 hours*
  - As blood glucose levels decrease, insulin levels decrease
  - *Respiratory quotient (RQ) decreases during starvation*
  - *Glucagon,* noradrenaline, cortisol, growth hormone, thyroxine levels *increase*
- 24 hours to 4 days
  - Gluconeogenesis increases from
    - *Amino acids due to breakdown of muscles, cause increased urinary output*
    - Glycerol from lipolysis
  - Gluconeogenesis happens in liver and kidney
  - Gluconeogenesis starts first followed by ketone bodies production leading to *metabolic acidosis*
  - One-third of brain requirements fulfilled by ketone bodies by day 3
- After 4 days
  - Transformation to ketone body production happens completely with the help of cortisol
  - Normal ketone levels: 0.2 mmol/L, starvation ketone level is 6-7 mmol/L
  - Red blood cells (RBCs), renal medulla and 50% of brain still needs glucose
  - Once fat deposits are over, death happens by protein malnutrition
- Body reserves
  - Glycogen: 0.5 kg, over in 24–48 hours

- o Lipids: 12–15 kg, over in 25 days
- o Proteins: 4–6 kg, over in 12 days
- Hypothermia: Hyperglycaemia, inhibition of coagulation cascade, left shift of oxyhaemoglobin dissociation curve (ODHC)
  - o Initially sinus bradycardia, at 30°C atrial irritability, <30°C ventricular fibrillation and asystole

Stress response to surgery

- Stress response: Derangements of metabolic and physiological processes in response to surgical trauma
- Response categories
  1. Neuroendocrine-metabolic response
  2. Inflammatory-immune response
- Neuroendocrine-metabolic response
  - o Sympathetic nervous system: *Adrenaline and noradrenaline* mobilise carbohydrate and fat stores and cause *hyperglycaemia*
  - o *Hypothalamic-pituitary-adrenal (HPA) axis*
    - • Cortisol is released and causes *hyperglycaemia*
  - o Growth hormone secretion: Hyperglycaemia
  - o Antidiuretic hormone (ADH; vasopressin): Water reabsorption
  - o Renin-angiotensin-aldosterone: Aldosterone causes *sodium and water reabsorption*
  - o Prolactin increases as well
- Inflammatory-immune response
  - o Cytokine release: Interleukin (IL)-1, IL-6, tumour necrosis factor (TNF)-α increase
  - o Acute phase response: C-reactive protein (CRP), fibrinogen, D-dimer increase
  - o Innate immune response: *Neutrophilia,* macrophages
- Phases of stress response
  - o The ebb phase: Initial period of shock when body is in shock and doesn't use any glucose that has become available due to mobilisation by stress response
  - o The catabolic phase: Period of protein and fat catabolism and weight loss
  - o The anabolic phase: Restoration of body protein and fat stores

- Modification of response by anaesthesia
  - **Propofol:** Blocks cortisol secretion
  - **Etomidate:** Blocks cortisol production. Inhibition of production continues for 6–12 hours after a single dose
  - **Volatile agents:** Inhibit adrenocorticotropic hormone (ACTH), cortisol, catecholamine and growth hormone secretion more than intravenous (IV) agents like propofol
  - **Benzodiazepines:** Inhibit cortisol production at the hypothalamic-pituitary level of the HPA axis
  - **α_2 Adrenergic agonists:** Block the sympathoadrenal and cardiovascular responses to a surgical stimulus
  - **Opioids:** High-dose opioids have been shown to completely suppress both ACTH and cortisol secretion
  - **Regional anaesthesia:** Blocks the endocrine and metabolic response to surgery

Blood

8

Blood

- The UK has the following percentage (%) of blood groups
  - O: 45%
  - A: 40%
  - B: 10%
  - AB: 5%
- A and B antigens (agglutinogens) are inherited as Mendelian dominants
- Rhesus factor has C, D and E antigens. D is the most antigenic; 85% of Caucasian population and 99% of the non-Caucasian population are D-rhesus positive

Storage of blood products

Component	Dose	Average bag	Temperature (Celsius)/ storage time
Packed red blood cells (RBCs)	1 bag increases haemoglobin (Hb) by 10g/L Children: mL = 0.5 × Wt (kg) × Hb (g/L) × (desired Hb – actual Hb)	300 mL	1–6°C/21–35 days
Fresh frozen plasma (FFP)	10–15 mL/kg	250 mL	–20°C/up to 1 year
Cryoprecipitate	Adult: 1 pool of cryoprecipitate increases fibrinogen by about 1 g/L (max 2 pools) or 1 unit/5–10 kg Children: 5–10 mL/kg	1 Unit: 10–15 mL Pooled product: 5 units	–20°C/up to 1 year
Platelets, apheresis	1 bag increases platelets by 30,000/μL Children: 5–10 mL/kg	300 mL	20–24°C/7–9 days

DOI: 10.1201/9781003390244-9

Prothrombin complex concentrate: Medication made up of blood clotting factors II, VII, IX and X. *Dose:* 25–50 units/kg for reversal of bleeding patient on warfarin. Consult haematologist for treatment and perioperative prophylaxis of haemorrhage in patients with congenital deficiency of factors II, VII, IX or X.

Storage Solutions

1. Acid-citrate-dextrose: 21 days
2. Citrate-phosphate-dextrose (CPD): 28 days
3. Citrate-phosphate-dextrose-adenine (CPDA): 35 days
4. Saline-adenine-glucose-mannitol (SAGM): 42 days

Blood transfusion reactions

Complications of blood transfusions

- **Febrile reactions (non-haemolytic reactions):** Recipient antibodies against donor white blood cell (WBC) antigens. Complement activation leads to ↑ interleukin (IL)-1, IL-6, tumour necrosis factor (TNF)-α
- **Haemolytic transfusion reactions:** ABO Incompatibility reaction. Recipient antibodies against donor antigens. Haemolysis → fever, disseminated intravascular coagulation (DIC), renal failure
- **Allergic reactions:** Allergic reaction to donor plasma proteins and can cause pruritus and urticaria
- **Transfusion-related acute lung injury (TRALI):** Donor antibodies against recipient WBC antigens. Acute respiratory distress syndrome (ARDS) within 6 hours of transfusion. More common in blood products with more plasma like fresh frozen plasma (FFP), platelets and cryoprecipitate
- **Transfusion-associated circulatory overload:** Respiratory distress due to pulmonary oedema like overload, hypertension, tachycardia and positive fluid balance
- **Infections:** HIV, hepatitis B, hepatitis C, malaria, syphilis, variant Creutzfeldt–Jakob disease (CJD), cytomegalovirus (CMV)
- **Graft vs host disease:** Very rare. Donor T-lymphocytes attack host bone marrow cells

Complications of massive blood transfusions

- Hypothermia
- Hyperkalaemia
- Hypocalcaemia
- Thrombocytopenia

- Coagulation factor depletion
- Metabolic alkalosis

Immunity

- Innate/Non-specific
  - **Barrier function:** Skin, gastric pH, lysozyme in sweat and tears
  - Complement system
  - **Neutrophils:** Phagocytosis
  - NK lymphocytes
  - **Macrophages:** Phagocytosis
  - **Eosinophils:** Helminths, parasites
- Acquired/Specific
  - Recognition of cells to be attacked
  - Delayed onset but powerful
  - Lymphocytes are the key cell
  - **Humoral:** Immunoglobins by plasma cells.
  - **Cellular:** T-lymphocytes
- T-lymphocytes
  - **Cytotoxic CD8:** Binds to T-cell receptor on major histocompatibility complex (MHC) class I and destroys the cell to which it is attached
  - **Helper CD4:** Binds to MHC class II on antigen-presenting cells
  - **Suppressor:** Negative feedback control
  - **Memory:** Proliferates cytotoxic cells on exposure
- Immunoglobins
  - **IgG:** Most abundant, fixes complement, only Ig that crosses the placenta
  - **IgA:** Secreted by epithelium
  - **IgM:** Largest antibody and first antibody that is secreted by the adaptive immune system
  - **IgD:** Antigen recognition by lymphocytes
  - **IgE:** Mast cell degranulation
- **Hypersensitivity:** Exaggerated immunologic responses occurring in response to an antigen
  - **Type I:** *Immediate* – IgE-mediated mast cell degranulation, e.g., anaphylaxis. Histamine release
  - **Type II:** *Cytotoxic* – Antibody-mediated cell lysis, e.g., transfusion reaction, Goodpasture's disease

- Type III: *Immune complex* – Deposition of antigen-antibody complexes causing local tissue damage, e.g., rheumatoid arthritis, systemic lupus erythematosus (SLE)
- Type IV: *Delayed* – Cell-mediated reaction by T-cells, e.g., Allergic contact dermatitis. Peripheral sensitisation of lymphocytes

If the patient has a history of anaphylaxis but doesn't know to which drug, and the case is non-urgent, postpone the case and try to get the notes from a previous hospital.

Complement system

- Enzyme system consisting of serum glycoproteins synthesised in liver involved in immunological processes
- Classical pathway
  - Antigen-antibody complex binds to C1
  - Activates C5
- Alternate pathway
  - Continuous and spontaneous activation by insoluble polysaccharides and foreign cells
  - Activates C5
- Common/Membrane attack pathway
  - C5 activation leads to binding of complement proteins (5b to 9) forming a complex which leads to lysis
- Functions of complement
  - C3a and C5a fragments: Release toxins that cause smooth muscle contraction, histamine release, increased vascular permeability
  - Complements C1, C2 and C3: Opsonisation
  - Membrane attack complex: Disrupts the cell membrane phospholipids to cause cell death

Coagulation system

- Coagulation system: Haemostasis between
  1. Endothelium
  2. Platelets
  3. Clotting factors

- **Endothelium**
  - Intact endothelium produces
    - **Antiplatelet:** Prostacyclin, nitric oxide (NO), ADPase
    - **Anticoagulants:** Heparin-like glycosaminoglycans, thrombomodulin (indirect thrombin inhibitor), tissue factor pathway inhibitor, tissue plasminogen activator (t-PA)
  - Damaged endothelium produces
    - Collagen, von Willebrand factor, tissue factor, plasminogen-activator inhibitor-1 (PAI-1)
- **Platelets**
  - **Adhesion:** von Willebrand factor
  - **Activation:** Factor V and VIII, calcium ions, thromboxane, ADP
  - **Aggregation:** GP IIb/IIIa receptor
- **Coagulation factors:** All clotting factors of formed by liver except factor VIII
- **Haemostasis:** Complex process that limits blood loss from damaged vessels
  - **Primary haemostasis:** Platelet deposition at the injury site
  - **Secondary haemostasis:** Plasma clotting factors leading to cross-linked fibrin
- **Anticoagulation pathway**
  1. **Fibrinolysis:** t-PA produced by endothelium converts. Plasminogen is converted into plasmin which turns fibrinogen into fibrinogen degradation products
  2. Tissue factor pathway inhibitor produced by endothelium
  3. **Proteins C and S:** Produced by liver. Inhibit thrombin and factor Va and VIIIa
  4. **Serine protease Inhibitors:** Antithrombin produced by liver. Inhibits thrombin and factors IXa, Xa, XIa, XIIa

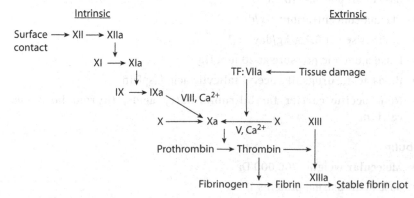

Figure 8.1   Classic cascade model.

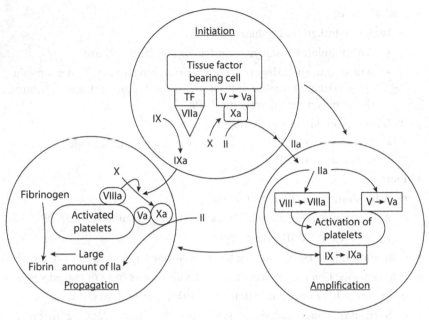

Figure 8.2 Cell-based model.

Plasma proteins

- **Plasma:** 5% of total body weight
- **Plasma proteins:** Albumin, all globulins except γ-globulins and fibrinogen synthesised in liver. γ-Globulins are synthesised in plasma cells

Albumin
- **Molecular weight: *65,000 Da***
- 65% of all plasma proteins
- **Plasma concentration:** 5 g/dL
- Synthesised at 0.2 g/kg/day
- Plasma oncotic pressure at 20 mm Hg
- Binds acidic drugs like acetyl salicylic acid (aspirin)
- Non-specific carrier for bilirubin, fatty acids, thyroid hormones, calcium

Globulin
- **Molecular weight:** 200,000 Da
- 35% of all plasma proteins

- Plasma concentration: 1.5 g/dL
- Plasma oncotic pressure at 5 mm Hg
- Types: α_1, α_2, β_1, β_2, γ subtypes
- α_1 Acid glycoprotein binds basic drugs like bupivacaine and angiotensinogen
- α_2 Globulins like haptoglobin bind free haemoglobin (Hb) released from haemolysis
- α_2 Globulins like ceruloplasmin bind copper
- β Globulins like transferrin bind iron in its Fe^{3+} form for transfer
- γ Globulins are antibodies produced by plasma cells

Fibrinogen

- Molecular weight: 350,000–500,000 Da
- 4% of all plasma proteins
- Plasma concentration: 0.5 g/dL
- Plasma oncotic pressure at 1 mm Hg

Regulatory proteins

- 1% of all plasma proteins
- Enzymes, proenzymes and hormones

Applied Physiology

9

Pregnancy

Parameter	Value changes
Cardiovascular system	
Cardiac output at first stage of labour	↑ 50%
Cardiac output at second stage of labour	↑ 60%
Cardiac output post-delivery	↑ 80–100%
Stroke volume	↑ 25–30%
Heart rate	↑ 15–25%
SVR	↓ 20%
PVR	↓ 35%
Intravascular fluid volume	↑ 35–45%
RBC volume	↑ 25%
Plasma volume	↑ 50%
CVP/PCWP	No change
Respiratory system	
Minute ventilation	↑ 45–50%
Respiratory rate	↑ 0–15%
Tidal volume	↑ 40–45%
Total lung capacity	↓ 0–5%
Vital lung capacity	No change
Functional residual capacity	↓ 20%
Residual volume	↓ 15–20%
FEV_1	No change
FEV_1/FVC	No change
Closing capacity	No change
Oxygen consumption	
At term	↑ 20%

(*Continued*)

DOI: 10.1201/9781003390244-10

Parameter	Value changes
At first stage of labour	↑ 40%
At second stage of labour	↑ 75%
Coagulation system	
Factors that increased	I, VII, VIII, IX, X, XII and vWF
Factors that decreased	XI, XIII, antithrombin III and tPA
Platelets	↓ 0–10%
Liver changes	
ALT/AST/Bilirubin	Increases to upper limit of normal
ALP	Double the normal level
Plasma cholinesterase	↓ 25–30%
Total protein	↓ 10%
Albumin	↓ 25%
Colloid osmotic pressure	27–22 mm Hg
Renal changes	
Renal blood flow	↑ 50–60%
GFR	↑ 50–60%
BUN	↓ 50%
Creatinine	↓ 50%
Arterial blood gases	
pH	7.42–7.44
$PaCO_2$	↓ to 30 mm Hg
PaO_2	More than 100 mm Hg
Bicarbonate	↓ to 20–21 mEq/L
Miscellaneous changes	
Leucocytes	Up to 13,000/mm^3
Minimum alveolar concentration	↓ 28%
Local anaesthetic sensitivity	Increases
Total thyroid hormones	↑
Thyroid-binding globulin	↑
Free T3 and T4	Unchanged

Increased venous return and hence increased plasma volume is the most important cause of increase oxygen flux during pregnancy.

Reduced intrathecal dose during pregnancy is due to engorgement of the epidural veins.

Fetal circulation

Vein/artery	Saturation (%)
Umbilical vein	80
IVC	65
SVC	25
Ascending aorta	60
Descending aorta	55
Pulmonary artery/Ductus arteriosus	50

Fetus	Adult
Ductus venosus	Ligamentum venosum
Ductus arteriosus	Ligamentum arteriosum
Left umbilical vein	Ligamentum teres
Left and right umbilical arteries	Umbilical ligaments
Foramen ovale	Fossa ovalis

- **Ductus arteriosus:** Closes when rise in arterial oxygen partial pressure causes vascular smooth muscle contraction. Closes in response to O_2. *Functional closure:* 24 hours. *Histological closure:* 3 weeks
- **Foramen ovale:** Closes when Left atrial pressure increases above right atrial pressure.
  Functional closure: At birth. *Histological closure:* 3–6 months
- **Ductus venosus:** *Closes last within 3–10 days*
- Only 10% of fetal blood enters pulmonary circulation
- Blood supply to the brain in foetus is more oxygenated than the rest of the body because blood from the right atrium is diverted through foramen ovale to the left atrium

Paediatrics

- A child under 16 years comes under the paediatrics definition
  - **Preterm:** Before 37 weeks, **Post-term:** After 42 weeks
  - **Neonate:** A baby up to 28 days or 44 weeks of age from date of conception
  - **Infants:** 1 month to 1 year
  - **Child:** 1–12 years
  - **Adolescent:** 13–16 years

- Airway
  - Large head, prominent occiput, short neck
  - Relatively large tongue compared with oral cavity
  - **High and anterior larynx:** Level of C3-4
  - Epiglottis is long, stiff and U-shaped
  - Larynx funnel-shaped and narrowest at cricoid
- Respiratory system
  - Horizontal ribs (prevent bucket-handle action)
  - Ventilation is mainly diaphragmatic
  - Low functional residual capacity (FRC)
  - Minute ventilation is rate dependent as tidal volume can't be increased
  - Closing volume larger than the FRC until 6–8 years of age
  - Work of respiration is 15% of oxygen consumption
  - **Oxygen consumption:** 7 mL/kg/min
  - Muscles of ventilation have low percentage of type 1 muscle fibres. Adult level by 1 year
  - 10% of total number of alveoli found in adults. Adult level by 8 years
  - Apnoea common in premature babies
- Cardiovascular system (CVS)
  - Dominant vagal tone
  - Cardiac output rate dependent
  - Cardiac output is 300–400 mL/kg/min at birth and 200 mL/kg/min during infancy
  - Blood volume
    - **Newborn:** 90 mL/kg
    - **Infant:** 85 mL/kg
- Renal system
  - Immature tubular function until 8 months
  - Low renal blood flow and glomerular filtration rate (GFR). Adult levels by 2 years
  - Extracellular fluid (ECF) is 40% of body weight
  - **Urine output:** 1–2 mL/kg/hr
- Neurological system
  - Can appreciate pain
  - Blood–brain barrier (BBB) is poorly formed
  - Cerebral regulation is present and functional from birth

- Hepatic system
  - Immature liver function
- Haematology
  - 70–90% of haemoglobin at birth is fetal haemoglobin (HbF)
  - HbF declines to 5% within 3 months
  - Haemoglobin at birth is 18–20 g/dL
  - Vitamin K-dependent clotting factors (II, VII, IX and X) and platelet function are deficient in the first few months
- Psychology
  - **Children less than 6 months:** Not upset by parent separation
  - **Children from 6 months to 4 years:** Upset by parent separation
- Preoperative fasting
  - **6 hours:** Solid
  - **4 hours:** Breast milk and formula feed
  - **2 hours:** Clear fluid
- Formulas
  - Weight (kg) = (age in years + 4) × 2
  - Endotracheal tube (ETT) size = age (years)/4 + 4
  - Length of ETT for correct placement
    - Oral = age (years)/2 + 12
    - Nasal = age (years)/2 + 15
  - **Systolic blood pressure (SBP; 50th centile mm Hg) from 1–15 years of age:** 90 + 2 × Age (years)
  - **Intraoperative maintenance fluid:** 4-2-1 formula. Isotonic fluids
  - **Fluid bolus in sepsis:** 20 mL/kg
  - **Fluid bolus in trauma:** 10 mL/kg
  - **Fluid bolus in circulatory failure:** 10 mL/kg
  - **Defibrillation dose:** 4 J/kg
- Midazolam, ketamine and clonidine are given as oral premedication as they are soluble in water and a small cup of clear liquid water can be given to reduce risk of aspiration
- Neonates have lower plasma proteins in serum compared with adults. Hence, free fraction of local anaesthetics is increased
- Atropine as premedication can cross BBB and cause confusion, tachycardia and mydriasis

Laparoscopy

- **Laparoscopy:** Peritoneal cavity insufflated at 4–6 L/min, maintained at constant gas flow of 200–400 mL/min. Benefits are
  - Less surgical trauma
  - Less postoperative pain
  - Less pulmonary dysfunction
  - Quicker recovery and shorter hospital stay
- **Physiologic changes**
  - **Respiratory system:** Atelectasis due to elevation of the diaphragm
    - ↓ Thoracopulmonary compliance by 30–50% and ↓ FRC
    - V/Q mismatched and increase in dead space and hypoxemia
    - CO_2 insufflation can cause pneumothorax, CO_2 subcutaneous emphysema, gas embolism and endobronchial intubation
  - **CVS system:** ↓ Cardiac output, ↑ systemic vascular resistance (SVR) and ↑ pulmonary vascular resistance
    - Heart rate remains unchanged or increases slightly
    - Lower limb venous stasis
    - Bradycardia due to peritoneal stretching and tachyarrhythmias due to ↑ CO_2
  - **Central nervous system (CNS):** An elevated intra-abdominal pressure (IAP) causes an increase in intracerebral pressure (ICP)
    - Prolonged steep Trendelenburg position increases the risk of cerebral oedema
  - **Gastrointestinal system:** Increase IAP can lead to ↑ risk for acid aspiration syndrome
    - Visceral and vascular damage can happen with blind trocar insertion
    - Persistent IAPs greater than 20 mm Hg will cause a reduction in mesenteric and gastrointestinal mucosal blood flow by up to 40%
    - Increased risk of postoperative nausea and vomiting (PONV)
  - **Renal system:** Urine output, renal plasma flow and GFR decrease to <50% of baseline values
    - Raised IAP has been recognised as an independent cause of acute kidney injury
  - **Problems with positioning: Common peroneal neuropathy,** meralgia paresthetica, femoral neuropathy can occur during **lithotomy position**
    - Brachial plexus injury can happen during positioning of hands over shoulders

- ◆ Steep Trendelenburg for laparoscopic prostatectomy can cause cerebral oedema
  - ○ Contraindications of laparoscopic surgery: It's never a low-risk procedure
    - ◆ Severe ischemic heart disease
    - ◆ Valvular disease
    - ◆ Significant renal dysfunction
    - ◆ End-stage respiratory disease

Prone position

- Prone position physiology
  - ○ **Respiratory system:** ↑ FRC, ↑ PaO_2, lung and chest wall compliance unchanged
    - ◆ More evenly distributed pulmonary blood flow, and improved V/Q matching
  - ○ **CVS system:** ↓ Cardiac output, ↓ stroke volume, little change in heart rate
    - ◆ Inferior vena cava (IVC) obstruction can cause increased bleeding from the vertebral venous plexus of Batson due to back pressure
  - ○ **CNS:** A rotated head position will reduce cerebral blood flow (CBF) and raise ICP
- Complications of prone positioning
  - ○ **Pressure injuries:** Either direct or indirect
    - ◆ **Direct injuries:** Skin necrosis, contact dermatitis, tracheal compression, salivary gland swelling, breast injury, injury to genitalia, compression of pinna and compression of the femoral neurovascular bundle
    - ◆ **Indirect injuries:** Macroglossia, mediastinal compression, visceral ischemia of liver and pancreas, avascular necrosis of femoral head, limb compartment syndrome and rhabdomyolysis
  - ○ **Ophthalmic complications**
    - ◆ Corneal abrasions
    - ◆ Subconjunctival haemorrhage
    - ◆ Central retinal artery occlusion
    - ◆ Ischemic optic neuropathy

- o Peripheral nervous system
  - ◆ Injury to ulnar nerve and brachial plexus
  - ◆ Injury to lateral cutaneous nerve of the thigh
- o Embolism
  - ◆ Venous gas embolism during posterior fossa cranial surgery

Elderly

- Elderly: >65 years of age
- CVS system: Cardiac output reduces by 3% per decade
  - o β adrenoreceptors in the myocardium are downregulated, less responsive to catecholamines
  - o Vascular system becomes less elastic, less compliant and less responsive to vasoconstricting drugs like metaraminol
  - o Postural hypotension is common
- Respiratory system: ↓ Total lung capacity (TLC), ↓ forced vital capacity (FVC), ↓ forced expiratory volume in 1 s (FEV$_1$)
  - o Residual volume (RV) and FRC remain unchanged
  - o By age of 65 years, closing capacity encroaches tidal volume
  - o Loss of elastic tissue around the oropharynx can lead to collapse of the airway
  - o Being edentulous makes bag mask ventilation difficult
- CNS: Neuronal density is reduced by 30% by the age of 80 years
  - o Visual and hearing impairment can lead to difficulty in communication
  - o Autonomic neuropathy can lead to hemodynamic instability
  - o Delirium (14–56%) is common in postoperative patients
- Renal system: GFR decreases by 1% per year over the age of 20 years
  - o Low muscle bulk, hence, low creatinine production, so even a small rise in creatinine level may indicate significant renal impairment
- Hepatic system: 20–40% decrease in liver blood flow with age
  - o Reduction in phase I drug metabolism
- Endocrine/metabolic: Basal metabolic rate falls by 1%/year after the age of 30
  - o 25% off patients over 85 years have non-insulin-dependent diabetes mellitus (NIDDM)

- **Musculoskeletal system:** Arthritis is common and can make regional anaesthesia techniques difficult
  - Thin skin and fragile subcutaneous blood vessels can make cannulation difficult
- **Pharmacology:** Minimal alveolar concentration (MAC) decreases by 6% per decade for all anaesthetics
  - Elderly patients have an increased sensitivity to CNS depressing drugs
  - Reduced cardiac output results in delayed onset of intravenous anaesthesia
  - Reduced total body water and increased adipose tissue leads
  - Plasma proteins are reduced leading to increased free drug availability
- **Frailty:** State of increased vulnerability to poor resolution of homeostasis after a stressor event. Frailty criteria
  - **Unintentional weight loss:** >10 pounds from baseline in prior year
  - **Reduced muscle strength:** Grip strength measured by a handheld dynamometer
  - **Exhaustion:** Feeling of exhaustion measured by a questionnaire
  - **Low physical activity:** Weekly kilocalorie consumption below the 20th percentile for their gender
  - **Slow walking:** A patient is timed to walk 15 feet. Time below the 20th percentile for their gender and height

Obesity

- **Obesity:** An individual with a body mass index (BMI) greater than 30 kg/m^2
- **World Health Organization (WHO) Classification for obesity**

BMI (kg/m²)		ASA grade
<18.5	Underweight	1
18.5–24.9	Normal weight	1
25–29.9	Overweight	1
>30	Obesity class 1	1
>35	Obesity class 2	2
>40	Obesity class 3	3

- Physiological changes
  - CVS: Ischemic heart disease, hypertension, cor pulmonale, venous thromboembolism
  - **Respiratory:** ↓ FRC, ↓ chest wall compliance, ↑ asthma, ↑ obstructive sleep apnoea (OSA),↑ pulmonary hypertension, chronic hypercarbia
  - **Metabolic:** ↑ diabetes mellitus (DM), ↑ fatty liver, ↑ gastroesophageal reflux disease (GERD), ↑ hiatal hernia
- **Drug dosing**

Lean body weight	Adjusted body weight	Total body weight
- Propofol induction - Non-depolarising NMBs - Paracetamol - Fentanyl - Alfentanil - Morphine - Local anaesthetics	- Propofol infusion - Antibiotics - Neostigmine (max 5 mg) - Sugammadex	- Suxamethonium - Low molecular weight heparin

- Lean body weight
- *Males maximum:* 100 kg, *Females maximum:* 70 kg
- Adjusted body weight: IBW + 40%
- Ideal body weight formula:
  - *Men:* 50 + 0.91 [*Height:* 152.4 cm]
  - *Women:* 45.5 + 0.91 [*Height:* 152.4 cm]

PHARMACOLOGY

General Pharmacology

10

Drug receptors

- **Receptors:** Proteins, either inside a cell or on its surface which receive a signal
- **Ligands:** A ligand is a substance that forms a complex with a receptor to serve a biological purpose
- Types of receptors
  - **Ligand-gated ion channel receptor**
    - Ion channel in cell membrane which opens directly after interaction with ligand
    - **For example, nicotinic acetylcholine receptor (NAChR):** Acetylcholine binds to two α subunits of the receptor to cause an influx of Na^+ ions causing depolarisation
    - **For example, $GABA_A$ receptor:** Benzodiazepines (BZDs) bind to receptors causing an influx of Cl^- ions
  - **G-protein–coupled receptor (GPCR)**
    - Channels in cell membrane coupled with G-protein to send secondary messengers to cause effect
    - For example, β adrenoreceptors and glucagon; G_s protein in membrane activates cAMP
    - For example, α_1 adrenoreceptor and muscarinic receptor; G_q-protein activates IP_3 and DAG
  - **Tyrosine kinase-linked receptor**
    - Membrane-bound receptors that mediate their effect by activating tyrosine kinase residues
    - **For example, insulin receptor:** Binding of insulin to the α subunit of receptor activates tyrosine kinase domains on each β subunit. The tyrosine kinase activity causes an autophosphorylation of several tyrosine residues in the β subunit
  - **Intracellular nuclear receptors**
    - Cytoplasmic receptors that mediate their effect by altering DNA transcription

DOI: 10.1201/9781003390244-12

- For example, thyroxine and steroid receptors: Hormones diffuse into cells and enter the nucleus. They interact with DNA to cause their effects over hours

G-proteins

- **GPCR:** Channels in cell membrane coupled with G-protein to send secondary messengers to cause signal transduction
- **Structure:** Seven α helix transmembrane domains that have an extracellular site for ligand binding and an intracellular site where G-protein attaches
- G-proteins are heterotrimeric proteins (α, β and γ subunits) which couple a surface receptor with an intracellular enzyme, e.g., cAMP leading to the required effect
- Types of G-proteins
  - G_s: β *adrenoreceptors and glucagon receptors* – G_s activates adenylate cyclase, adenylate cyclase helps create more cAMP and cAMP activates protein kinase A
  - G_i: α_2 *adrenoreceptors and opioid receptors* – G_i inactivates adenylate cyclase. Decrease in adenylate cyclase causes reduced levels of cAMP. Low levels of cAMP lead to a decrease in levels of protein kinase A
  - G_q: α_1 *adrenoreceptors and muscarinic acetylcholine receptors (mAChRs)* – G_q activation causes increase in phospholipase C (PLC). Increase in PLC leads to increased breakdown of PIP_2 into IP_3, which causes increased calcium release from endoplasmic reticulum and DAG, which activates protein kinase C
- **Secondary messengers:** A molecule that is released intracellularly as part of signal transduction pathway after activation of a cell surface receptor, e.g., Ca^{2+}
- Mechanism of action of GPCR
  - Ligand binds to the extracellular site of GPCR. GPCR has an intracellular $\alpha\beta\gamma$ heterotrimeric unit as well. This ligand binding causes the intracellular α subunit to attach to a GTP molecule
  - Intracellular $\beta\gamma$ units dissociate from the α-GTP complex, which activates or inhibits enzyme systems like guanylate cyclase, resulting in production of secondary messengers
  - The α subunit with its intrinsic GTPase activity breaks down GTP into GDP and P_i
  - The α-GDP complex releases α subunit and GDP. The α subunit rejoins $\beta\gamma$ subunits to return to the resting unit

Secondary messengers

Receptor transducer	Receptor type	Effect
G_s	- Adrenoreceptor ($\beta_{1,2,3}$) - Serotonin (5-HT$_{4,6,7}$) - Dopamine (D$_1$, D$_5$) - Histamine (H$_2$) - Adenosine (A$_2$)	$\uparrow$ Adenylyl cyclase $\downarrow$ $\uparrow$ cAMP $\downarrow$ $\uparrow$ Protein kinase A
G_i	- Adrenoreceptor (α_2) - Muscarinic (M$_2$, M$_4$) - Serotonin (5-HT$_{1,5}$) - Dopamine (D$_2$) - Adenosine (A$_1$, A$_3$) - Opioids (μ, K, δ)	$\downarrow$ Adenylyl cyclase $\downarrow$ $\downarrow$ cAMP $\downarrow$ $\downarrow$ Protein kinase A
G_q	- Adrenoreceptor (α_1) - Muscarinic (M$_1$, M$_3$, M$_5$) - Serotonin (5-HT$_2$) - Histamine (H$_1$)	Phospholipase C $\downarrow$ PIP$_2$ $\downarrow$ IP$_3$ + DAG $\downarrow$ $\downarrow$ $\uparrow$ Ca^{2+} protein kinase C

Chemical	Receptor
Insulin Prolactin	Tyrosine Kinase Receptors
ADH Glucagon Salbutamol Theophylline	$\uparrow$ cAMP
NO ANP	$\uparrow$ cGMP

Drug action

- Receptors
  - Ligand-gated ion channel receptor
    - **For example, nAChR:** Acetylcholine binds to two α subunits of the receptor to cause an influx of Na$^+$ ions causing depolarisation

- ○ GPCR
  - ✦ For example, β adrenoreceptors and glucagon; G_s protein in membrane activates cAMP
- ○ Tyrosine kinase-linked receptor
  - ✦ For instance, insulin receptor at insulin receptor
- ○ Intracellular nuclear receptors
  - ✦ For example, thyroxine hormone at thyroid receptor
- **Ion channels**
  - ○ Lidocaine acts upon and blocks the fast Na^+ channel
- **Enzymes**
  - ○ Aspirin inhibits cyclooxygenase enzyme
- **Hormones**
  - ○ Sulfonylureas increase insulin release
- **Neurotransmitters**
  - ○ Amitriptyline reduces noradrenaline reuptake
- **Transport systems**
  - ○ Furosemide blocks $Na^+/K^+/2Cl^-$ ATPase pump in the loop of Henle
- **Physicochemical**
  - ○ Sugammadex chelates rocuronium

Drug interactions

- **Drug interaction:** When a drug's mechanism of action is disturbed by the concomitant administration of another drug
- **Classification:** Physicochemical, pharmacodynamic, pharmacokinetic
- **Physicochemical:** Interactions due to physical properties of the drugs themselves
  - ○ **Chelation:** Deferoxamine and iron, sugammadex and rocuronium
  - ○ **Neutralisation:** Antacids are bases that neutralize the acid made in the stomach
  - ○ **Precipitation:** Thiopentone can precipitate with either pancuronium or vecuronium
  - ○ **Adsorption:** Halothane and rubber tubes
- **Pharmacodynamic:** Interactions when action of one drug is affected by the action of another drug
  - ○ **Summation:** When action of both drugs is additive and equal to sum of individual drugs, e.g., propofol and midazolam, inhalational agents and N_2O

- o **Synergism:** When action of both drugs is additive and greater than the sum of individual drugs, e.g., trimethoprim and sulfamethoxazole, propofol and remifentanil
- o **Potentiation:** When action of one drug is amplified by the addition of another drug, e.g., neuromuscular blockers and magnesium; probenecid decreases renal excretion of penicillin and increases its levels in body
- o **Antagonism:** Action of one drug is blocked by another drug, e.g., BZD by flumazenil, morphine by naloxone
- **Pharmacokinetic:** When one drug alters the way the body handles the other drug
  - o **Absorption:** Adrenaline reduces the absorption of lidocaine by causing vasoconstriction and prolongs its action
  - o **Distribution:** Non-steroidal anti-inflammatory drugs (NSAIDs) displace warfarin from plasma proteins, increasing free warfarin levels, thus, increasing chances of bleeding
  - o **Metabolism:** Barbiturates induce hepatic enzymes increasing metabolism of drugs
  - o **Excretion:** Alkalinisation of urine to increase excretion of salicylates

Drug bioavailability

- **Bioavailability:** Fraction of the drug that enters the bloodstream. Hence, 100% of intravenous drugs
- **Oral bioavailability:** Area under the concentration-time curve (AUC) of drug administered orally to AUC of drug administered intravenously
- **First-pass metabolism: The degree of metabolism of an orally administered drug that occurs in liver before it reaches systemic circulation**

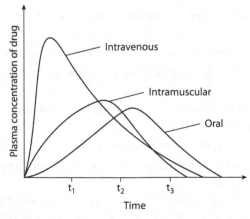

Figure 10.1 Bioavailability.

- Drugs with high first-pass metabolism
  - Morphine, aspirin, diazepam
- **Factors affecting drug absorption**
  - Route of administration
  - pKa and ionisation
  - Lipid solubility
  - Particle size
  - Regional blood flow
  - Protein binding
- **Acidic drugs:** Salicylic acid pKa 3, frusemide pKa 3.9, thiopentone pKa 7.6, paracetamol pKa 9.5, propofol pKa 11
- **Basic drugs:** Diazepam pKa 3.7, etomidate pKa 4.1, ketamine pKa 7.5, bupivacaine pKa 8.2, morphine pKa 8.6
- **Paraldehyde** is an anticonvulsant given most commonly per rectal in children for status epilepticus

Isomerism

- **Isomerism:** Molecules that have the same molecular formula, same molecular weight but different structural arrangement and, hence, different chemical and physical properties
- **Classification:** A, structural isomers; B, stereoisomers
- **Structural isomer:** Same molecular formula but different chemical formula
  - **Chain isomers:** Carbon skeleton changes but functional group remains in the same position, e.g., butane and isobutene
  - **Position isomers:** Carbon skeleton stays the same but functional group varies position, e.g., isoflurane and enflurane
  - **Functional isomers:** Carbon skeleton stays the same but functional group changes, e.g., acetaldehyde and acetone
  - **Tautomers:** Molecule exists in two different forms depending upon the physiochemical environment around it. Midazolam exists in open ring structure in pH <4 and closed ring structure in pH >4
- **Stereoisomers:** Same molecular formula and chemical formula but different spatial arrangements
  - **Enantiomers (optical isomers):** Molecules with a single chiral centre form mirror images of each other, but these images can't be superimposed upon each other. Nomenclature can be
    - **Dextro and laevorotatory:** Rotate polarised light in right or left direction. Abbreviated as (*d*) and (*l*) or (+) and (−). Old classification

- ◆ **D and L prefixes (Fischer–Rosanoff convention):** Orientation of atomic structure of sugar and amino acid structure in the molecule, e.g., look for the OH group of the asymmetric carbon. If it's located on the right, we designate it with D, and vice versa. Structural definition, not related to optical properties
- ◆ **Rectus (R) and Sinister (S):** Reflects the direction of ascending atomic number of the atoms attached to the chiral centre. Counting done from highest to lowest atomic number. If number descends in a clockwise direction, isomer is the R form and vice versa, for example, levobupivacaine and S-bupivacaine, ketamine and S-ketamine
  - ○ **Diastereoisomers:** Molecules with more than one chiral centre, e.g., atracurium has four chiral centres
  - ○ **Cis-trans isomers (geometric isomers):** Molecules have a double bond around which the atoms can't rotate, e.g., mivacurium
    - ◆ **Cis-form:** Groups on same side
    - ◆ **Trans-form:** Groups on opposite sides

Adverse drug reactions

- **Adverse drug reactions (ADRs):** Unintended, harmful reactions to medicines
- ADRs have been classified into type A and type B
- **Type A**
  - ○ Dose dependent
  - ○ Predictable due to known pharmacology
  - ○ Common
  - ○ High morbidity but low mortality
- **Type B**
  - ○ Idiosyncratic and bizarre
  - ○ Unpredictable
  - ○ Uncommon
  - ○ Low morbidity but high mortality
  - ○ **Anaphylactic reaction:** IgE mediated, **histamine release**
  - ○ **Anaphylactoid reaction:** Non-IgE mediated
- **World Health Organization (WHO) classification**
  - ○ **Augmented:** Dose related
  - ○ **Bizarre:** Non-dose related

- ○ **Chronic:** Dose and time related
- ○ **Delayed:** Time related
- ○ **End of use:** Withdrawal
- ○ **Failure:** Treatment failure
- **Porphyrinogens**
  - ○ Thiopentone
  - ○ Ketamine
  - ○ Etomidate
  - ○ Midazolam

Drug metabolism by liver

- **Drug metabolism reactions in liver:** In smooth reticulum of liver
  - ○ **Phase I reactions:** Oxidation, reduction or hydrolysis of the drug
    - ◆ Cytochrome P450 enzyme is involved
  - ○ **Phase II reactions:** Glucuronidation, sulphation, acetylation and methylation
    - ◆ They increase solubility of the drugs
- **Drugs metabolised by cytochrome P 450 system**

Inducers	Inhibitors
Barbiturates	Etomidate
Phenytoin	Ciprofloxacin
Carbamazepine	Erythromycin
Glucocorticoids	Fluconazole
Rifampicin	Metronidazole
Acute alcohol intake	Chronic alcohol intake
Smoking	Grapefruit
	Cimetidine
	Amiodarone

- **Effect of chronic liver disease on drugs used in anaesthesia**
  - ○ Hepatic clearance based upon blood flow to liver and drugs unbound to plasma proteins
  - ○ Drugs with low extraction ratios, less than 0.3. Metabolism affected by protein bounding and not by liver blood flow

- o Drugs with high extraction ratios, greater than 0.7. Metabolism affected by liver blood flow
- o Induction agents like etomidate and **propofol are highly lipophilic and have high extraction ratios.** Elimination is prolonged but redistribution is not. Pharmacodynamic effects are enhanced and duration of action is increased
- o BZDs and **thiopental have low extraction ratios.** Unbound drug increases because of low protein synthesis. This leads to a pronounced effect
- o Opioid metabolism is decreased in liver disease, specifically the ones that are metabolised by liver like morphine and pethidine. They have an enhanced pharmacodynamic effect. Remifentanil metabolised by esterases is not affected by liver disease
- o Neuromuscular blocking agents like vecuronium and rocuronium metabolised by liver are prolonged in their action. Action of atracurium and cis-atracurium is not prolonged. Effect of suxamethonium is prolonged as plasma cholinesterase decreases

Drug metabolism in kidneys

- • **Drug handling by kidneys**
  - o **Glomerular filtration:** Smaller molecules (<60,000 Da) are readily filtered. Highly protein-bound drugs are not readily filtered
  - o **Proximal tubular secretion:** Two types of carrier exist
    - ◆ **Acidic drugs:** NSAIDs, penicillin and furosemide
    - ◆ **Alkaline drugs:** Dopamine
    - ◆ Tubular secretion is active carrier medicated and can transport drugs against their concentration gradient
  - o **Distal tubular reabsorption:** Passive as water is reabsorbed along the tubule, drug concentration increases in lumen and gets reabsorbed
    - ◆ Highly lipid soluble drugs like fentanyl are reabsorbed in circulation
    - ◆ Changes in urine pH change the tubular reabsorption. Sodium bicarbonate is used to alkalinize overdose of aspirin
- • **Effect of chronic kidney disease (CKD) on drugs used in anaesthesia**
  - o Inhalational agents, except methoxyflurane and enflurane, are not affected by kidney disease metabolically
  - o Thiopental has reduced protein binding in CKD. Therefore, clinical effects are exaggerated
  - o **Propofol is metabolised mostly by the liver mostly; thus, end-stage renal disease (ESRD) doesn't increase its effect**

○ Ketamine is less protein bound and is mostly metabolised by liver, hence, less affected by CKD

○ Etomidate though, like thiopental, is 75% protein bound, and its effects are not increased by CKD

○ BZDs are highly protein bound and their effect is increased by CKD due to increased free fraction

○ Opioids like **morphine and pethidine have prolonged effects.** *Fentanyl, alfentanil and remifentanil are better choices in CKD*

○ Muscle relaxants like atracurium and cis-atracurium are not affected by CKD. Suxamethonium with CKD can cause dangerous hyperkalaemia

○ Sugammadex is not approved for use in patients with ESRD

○ **Labetalol is metabolised in liver and ranitidine is excreted unchanged in urine**

Dose-response curves

- **Potency:** A measure of the quantity of the drug needed to produce maximal effect. The smaller the dose, more potent is the drug

- **Efficacy:** Ability of a drug to produce the maximal response once the drug is bound, e.g., *morphine with 100% intrinsic activity at the mu opioid receptor*

- **Affinity:** A measure of how keenly a drug binds to a receptor

- ED_{50}: Dose of a drug required to produce 50% of its maximum effect

- EC_{50}: Concentration of a drug required to produce 50% of its maximal effect

- LD_{50}: Dose of a drug required to produce a lethal effect in 50% of sample population

- **Full agonist:** Has affinity to receptor and efficacy = 1, e.g., morphine

- **Partial agonist:** Has affinity to receptor and efficacy <1, e.g., buprenorphine

- **Inverse agonist:** Has affinity to receptor, but effect is the exact opposite to that of the endogenous ligand. Efficacy = –1, e.g., naloxone

- **Antagonist:** Has affinity to receptor but has no effect of its own. Efficacy = 0. It stops agonists from doing their own action, e.g., esmolol on β adrenoreceptors

- **Competitive antagonist:** Binds to receptor on the same site as agonist, and antagonism can be prevented by increasing the dose of agonist. For example, rocuronium competing with acetylcholine at the NAChR

- **Non-competitive antagonist:** Binds to receptor on a different site as agonist, and antagonism can't be prevented by increasing the dose of agonist, e.g., ketamine on N-methyl-D-aspartate (NMDA) receptor

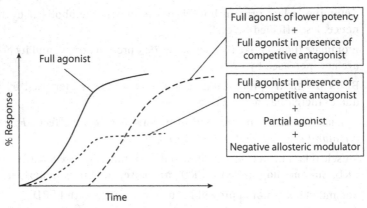

Figure 10.2 Semi-logarithmic dose-response curves.

Elimination kinetics

- **Volume of distribution (V_d):** Theoretical volume of fluid into which the total amount of drug administered reaches following its administration
  - The V_d may exceed the total body water volume due to drug tissue binding. Highly lipid-soluble drugs like fentanyl have a large V_d 4L/kg
- **Elimination:** Irreversible removal of drug from the body after distribution, metabolism or excretion
  - To maintain a desired plasma concentration of a drug at steady state, the rate of elimination must equal the rate of administration
- **Clearance:** The theoretical volume of plasma from which a drug is removed per unit time (mL/min)
  - Liver and kidney disease can affect metabolism and excretion of disease and, hence, decrease clearance
- **First-order kinetics:** *Constant proportion of the drug is administered*
  - Clearance and half-life can be used to describe elimination kinetics
  - Rate of elimination varies
  - **Exponential process**
  - Non-saturable enzymes
- **Zero-order kinetics:** *Constant amount of drug is eliminated*
  - Clearance and half-life can't be used to describe elimination kinetics
  - Rate of elimination is constant
  - Enzymes saturated
  - For example, alcohol, phenytoin, thiopentone and theophylline

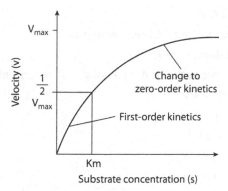

Figure 10.3 Michaelis–Menten graph.

- **Half-life:** Time taken for plasma concentration of a drug to reduce to half its original value
  - After five half-lives, elimination is 96.875% complete
- **Time constant:** The time taken for plasma concentration of a drug to fall to 37% of its original value
  - The time that would be taken for the initial concentration to fall to zero if the initial rate of decline continues

Drug	Alfentanil	Fentanyl
Dose	5–25 µg/kg	1–2 µg/kg
Duration of action	10 mins	30 mins
Lipid solubility	+	+++
pKa	6.5	8.4
Percentage un-ionised	90%	9%
V_d	4 L/kg	0.8 L/kg
Clearance	300-500 mL/min	500–1500 mL/min
$T_{1/2}$	120 mins	360 mins

Formulas used in general pharmacology

- **Volume of distribution:** V_d = Initial dose/C_o
  where C_o is plasma concentration at time zero
- **Clearance:** $Cl = V_d \times k_e$
  where k_e is elimination rate constant (1/min)
- **Clearance:** $Cl = Dose/AUC$
  where AUC is the area under the concentration-time curve

- **Clearance:** $Cl = Q/ER$

  where Q is flow rate and ER is extraction ratio

- **Rate of elimination:** $E = Cl \times C_{ss}$

  where C_{ss} is plasma concentration at steady state (mg/mL)

- **Time constant:** $\tau = 1/k_e$

- **Time constant:** $\tau = V_d/Cl$

- **Half-life:** $t_{1/2} = 0.693\tau$

- **Half-life:** $t_{1/2} = 0.693/k_e$

- **Michaelis–Menten equation:**

$$V = V_{max} [S]/K_m + [S]$$

where V is the velocity of reaction, V_{max} is the maximum velocity of reaction, K_m is the Michaelis constant and [S] is the concentration of substrate

Alveolar pressure (P) of an inhalation agent at concentration (c) at Time (t) with the constant (k)

$$P = ce^{-kt}$$

Compartment models

- **Compartment models:** They predict the distribution of a drug after administration
- **Single compartment:** Drug given enters a single compartment only
  - The volume of this compartment C1 is the total volume of distribution
  - The central compartment will be called C1
  - Rate constant for a drug moving from outside to central compartment is K_{01}
  - Rate constant for a drug being eliminated from central compartment is K_{10}
  - Non-physiological. Used for aminoglycoside concentrations

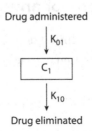

Drug administered

K_{01}

C_1

K_{10}

Drug eliminated

Figure 10.4 One-compartment model.

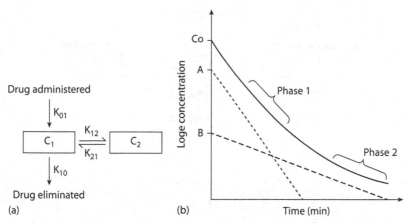

Figure 10.5 (a and b) Two-compartment model.

- **Two-compartment model:** Total of two compartments, one central and one less vascular peripheral compartment like muscle
  - The central compartment will be called C1. Peripheral compartment will be called C2
  - The total volume of compartments C1 + C2 is the total volume of distribution
  - K_{12} represents drug movement from C1 to C2 and K_{21} is from C2 to C1
  - Elimination occurs only from central compartment
  - Phase 1 shows distribution of drug from C1 to C2 and phase 2 shows elimination from C1
  - Used for thiopentone and vancomycin concentrations
- **Three-compartment model:** A third least vascular compartment like fat is added to the previous two compartments
  - The central compartment will be called C1. Peripheral compartment will be called C2. It has rapid equilibrium with C1. The third compartment will be called C3 and has slow equilibrium with central compartment C1
  - The total volume of compartments C1 + C2 + C3 is the total volume of distribution
  - K_{13} represents drug movement from C1 to C3 and K_{31} is from C3 to C1
  - Elimination still occurs only from the central compartment
  - Phase 1 shows distribution of drug from C1 to C2, phase 2 shows distribution of drug from C1 to C3 and phase 3 shows elimination from C1
  - Used for target-controlled infusion (TCI) algorithms for total intravenous anaesthesia (TIVA), e.g., propofol, remifentanil

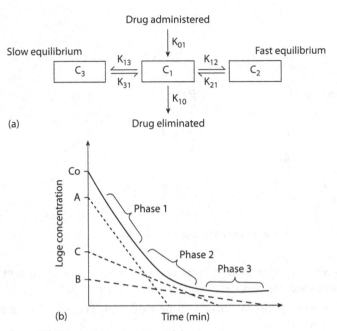

(a)

(b)   Time (min)

Figure 10.6   (a and b) Three–compartment model.

Context sensitive half-time

- **Context sensitive half-time (CSHT):** Time taken for plasma concentration to halve after an infusion to maintain blood levels is stopped
  - Context here is that the half-time will vary with the duration of drug infusion

Drug	CSHT after 2 hours of infusion	CSHT after 8 hours of infusion
Propofol	16 mins	41 mins
Remifentanil	4.5 mins	9 mins
Fentanyl	48 mins	282 mins
Alfentanil	50 mins	64 mins

- When an infusion is stopped, the drug will continue to move down a concentration gradient into the second and third compartments until equilibrium occurs among all three compartments
  - The drug will also be metabolised from the central compartment
  - Metabolism leads to a reduction in plasma concentration and, hence, reduce concentration in the central compartment

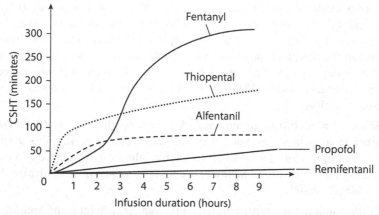

Figure 10.7   Context-sensitive half-time.

○ Now a reverse concentration gradient and drug goes from peripheral tissue to central compartment

○ This leads to maintenance of plasma concentration well beyond the end of the infusion

Alfentanil can be used for TIVA over fentanyl for a short duration surgery because of rapid offset of alfentanil due to small volume of distribution.

Alfentanil has a faster onset of action than fentanyl due to having a lower pKa than fentanyl.

Target-controlled infusions (TCIs)

- TCIs: Infusions that use a pharmacokinetic mathematical model generated by a microprocessor-driven pump to maintain a pre-defined target plasma concentration
- They use three-compartment models to predict plasma and effect site concentration of the drug
- A bolus/elimination/transfer (BET) principle is used to quantify plasma level of a drug
  ○ V1 is the central compartment that is filled by a bolus. V2 is the rapidly equilibrating compartment. V3 is the slowly equilibrating compartment
  ○ Bolus (B) fills the central compartment. Infusion given at a rate of elimination rate (E) plus redistribution rate to the peripheral compartment (T)

- **Marsh model:** Used for propofol. Weight of patient is entered, and age is ignored. Used for age >16 years only. Hence, the volume of V1 (Marsh 19.4 L vs Schnider 4.27 L for an 85 kg individual) is four times the volume in the Schnider model. Hence, a bigger bolus is given initially even in an older patient. The original Marsh model targeted only plasma concentrations. A modified Marsh model is used now which uses effect site concentration

- **Schnider model:** Used for propofol. Age, sex, height and weight are combined to ascertain lean body mass. A fixed volume of 4.27 L is used as V1. The bolus can thus be small in overweight patients and be clinically inadequate. Overall, the Schnider model is more accurate clinically than the Marsh model

- **Minto model:** Used with remifentanil. Age, sex, height and weight are combined to ascertain lean body mass. A fixed volume of 5.42 L is used as V3

- **Kataria model:** The Kataria model is validated for use in patients aged 3–16 years with a minimum weight of 15 kg

- **Paedfusor model:** The Paedfusor model is used for patients 1–16 years of age

- **Eleveld model:** This model does not use lean body mass. Can be used in all patients aged 27 weeks to 88 years. Validated until 200 kg compared with 160 kgs for the Schnider model. The covariates in Eleveld are height, weight, sex, age and the presence or absence of concomitant analgesic drugs (remifentanil). Can be used for providing both anaesthetic and sedative concentrations of propofol

- **When using TIVA, secure vascular access is the most important mechanism to avoid awareness**

Anaesthetic Pharmacology

11

Meyer–Overton hypothesis and MAC

- Minimum alveolar concentration (MAC_{50}) defines the anaesthetic depth for inhaled agents at which 50% of patients respond to painful stimulus with movement
  - MAC-awake: MAC at which eyes open to verbal command during emergence from anaesthesia. 0.3-0.4 MAC
  - MAC-bar: MAC blocks autonomic responses to surgical incision in 50% of patients. 1.5 MAC
- Potency: *Described by oil:* Gas partition coefficient. *Higher the oil:* Gas partition coefficient, the more potent the gas
- Onset/Offset of anaesthesia: *Described by blood:* Gas partition coefficient. *Lower the blood:* Gas solubility, faster is onset of action
  - *Blood/gas partition coefficient:* Dimensionless number. Ratio of solubility of anaesthetic in blood and gas
- Meyer–Overton hypothesis states that once enough number of volatile agents were dissolved in lipid membranes of brain cells, anaesthesia would start. So direct correlation between lipid solubility (*oil: gas partition coefficient*) and potency (MAC)
- If the theory was right then the *product of oil: gas partition coefficient* and MAC would be constant. But that is not the case with newer inhalational agents

MAC increased by	MAC decreased by
Hyperthermia	Hypothermia
Hypercapnia	Hypocapnia
Hypernatremia	Hyponatremia
Increasing age	Decreasing age
Chronic alcohol	Acute alcohol/central nervous system (CNS) sedatives (Clonidine, methyldopa)

(Continued)

DOI: 10.1201/9781003390244-13

MAC increased by	MAC decreased by
Thyrotoxicosis	Hypothyroid
Severe anxiety	Severe anaemia
Increase in ambient pressure	Pregnancy
Cocaine/Amphetamines	Opioids/Lithium

- MAC not affected by haemoglobin concentration, neostigmine (doesn't cross blood–brain barrier [BBB]) and magnesium concentration.

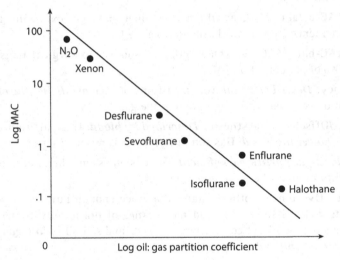

Figure 11.1 Potency vs lipid solubility.

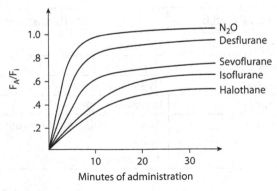

Figure 11.2 Wash-in curve.

Inhalational agents

	Halothane	Isoflurane	Sevoflurane	Desflurane	N$_2$O	Xenon
Molecular weight	197	184	200	168	44	131
Blood:gas	2.4	1.4	0.7	0.42	0.47	0.14
Oil:gas	224	98	80	29	1.4	1.9
MAC (%)	0.75	1.17	1.8	6.6	105	71
% Metabolised (liver microsomes)	20	0.2	3.5	0.02	0.01	Nil
Boiling point (°C)	50	48.5	58.5	23.5	−88	−108
Saturated vapour pressure (SVP) at 20°C (kPa)	32.3	33.2	22.7	89.2	5200	N/A
Odour	Non-irritant	Irritant	Non-irritant	Pungent	Odour-less	Odour-less

- Cigarette smoking doesn't affect choice of anaesthetic
- Halothane: Only halothane contains bromine atoms
  - *Reversible transaminitis* due to hepatic hypoxia
  - Fulminant hepatitis: After repeated use. Immune response to production of trifluoroacetylated proteins which bind to liver
  - Prepared with thymol 0.01% to prevent 0.01% to prevent decomposition due to light exposure
- Isoflurane
  - Coronary steal: In the presence of stenoses this may steal blood away from ischaemic endocardium
- Sevoflurane: Denser than air
  - Produces compounds A–E when interacting with soda lime. Compound A causes hepatic, renal and central nervous system (CNS) toxicity in rats, but is not known to cause toxicity in humans

- **Desflurane**
  - Stimulates sympathetic nervous system causing tachycardia and hypertension
  - Requires special vaporiser (pressurised at 2 atm, 39°C) due to extreme volatility

	Halothane	Isoflurane	Sevoflurane	Desflurane	N_2O
Respiratory rate	↑	↑↑	↑↑	↑↑	↑
Tidal volume	↓	↓↓	↓	↓↓	↓
$PaCO_2$	±	↑↑	↑	↑↑	±
Bronchodila-tion	Yes			Irritant	±
Contractility	↓↓↓	↓	↓	±	↓
Heart rate	↓↓	↑↑	±	↑ (↑↑ > 1.5 MAC)	±
Systemic vascular resistance	↓	↓↓	↓	↓↓	±
Blood pressure	↓↓	↓↓	↓	↓↓	±
Sensitivity to catechol-amines	↑↑↑	±	±	±	±
Cerebral blood flow	↑↑↑	↑ (Yes MAC > 1)	Preserves autoregula-tion	↑	↑
Cerebral O_2 requirement	↓	↓	↓	↓	↑
Electroen-cephalogra-phy (EEG)	Burst suppression	Burst suppression	Burst suppression	Burst suppression	Slows delta oscillations
Uterus	Some relaxation				±
Muscle relaxation	Some	Significant	Significant	Significant	±
Analgesia	Some analgesia				Good analgesia

To increase end–tidal inhalational concentration during low flow anaesthesia, the quickest option is to increase the fresh gas flow.

Nitrous oxide

- Production: Ammonium nitrate heated at 240°C. $NH_4NO_3 \rightarrow N_2O + 2H_2O$
  - Impurities like NH_3, N_2 and NO_2 are removed prior to storage
- Physiochemical properties
  - Critical temperature: 36.5°C
  - Critical pressure: 72 bar
  - Boiling point: –88°C
  - Blood gas partition coefficient: 0.47
  - Oil gas partition coefficient: 1.4
  - A normal N_2O cylinder will show gauge pressure of 44 bar until it is nearly empty
- Mechanism of action
  - Inhibits N-methyl-D-aspartate (NMDA) receptors
  - Stimulation of dopaminergic neurons, mediates release of endogenous opioids
- Pharmacodynamic actions
  - **Cardiovascular system (CVS):** Myocardial contractility decreases; however, blood pressure remains unchanged
  - **Respiratory:** Tidal volume decreases but respiratory rate increases, hence, minute ventilation is unchanged
  - **CNS:** Increases cerebral O_2 requirement and cerebral blood flow
  - **Concentration effect:** N_2O is 25 times more soluble than N_2 in blood so it diffuses faster than N_2 in blood. Thus, remaining gases like inhalational agents are increased in alveoli, which is known as *concentration effect*
  - **Second gas effect:** As concentration gradient of inhalational agents between alveoli and blood increases, there is faster diffusion of other gases into blood and, hence, faster onset of anaesthesia, which is known as *second gas effect. It applies during extubation as well with patients having higher N_2O recovering earlier*
- Side effects
  - **Postoperative nausea and vomiting:** Bowel distension and opioid effects
  - **Diffusion hypoxia:** After discontinuation of nitrous oxide, concentration gradient between the gases in the alveoli and blood reverses rapidly. Now N_2O fills the alveoli more rapidly diluting oxygen in alveoli causing hypoxia. This can be prevented by 100% oxygen following N_2O cessation
  - **Expansion of nitrogen-containing cavities:** As N_2O is 25 times more soluble than N_2 in blood, it diffuses quicker than N_2 from blood in these cavities. Thus, it can increase pressure in air-filled cavities like

middle ear, bowel, pneumothorax and eye filled with gas such as SF_6 after vitreoretinal surgery

- o **Bone marrow and neurotoxicity:** N_2O oxidizes the cobalt atom of the vitamin B_{12} complex. Vitamin B_{12} acts as a cofactor for methionine synthetase. Hence, N_2O blocks methionine synthetase. Methionine is a precursor to the S-adenosyl methionine (SAM), which is incorporated into myelin. Absence of myelin leads to subacute combined systems degeneration of the cord. Methionine is also a precursor of tetrahydrofolate, which is important for DNA synthesis needed for red blood cell (RBC) production. Hence N_2O can cause megaloblastic anaemia

- o **Greenhouse effect:** N_2O is 300 times more potent than CO_2 in its potential to trap atmospheric heat. Anaesthesia gases contribute to about 1% of global total

- **Clinical uses**
  - o Used in general anaesthesia to reduce the amount of volatile gas use and faster onset of action in children
  - o Entonox (N_2O:O_2::50:50) is used for analgesia in pregnant females

Intravenous induction agents

	Propofol	Thiopental	Etomidate	Ketamine
Chemical	2.6 Diisopropylphenol	Sulphur analogue of oxybarbiturate	Imidazole derivative	Phencyclidine derivative
Presentation	- 1% or 2% emulsion (not soluble in water) - 10% Soyabean oil - 1.2% Purified egg phosphatide - 2.25% Glycerol	- 2.5% Sodium salt - Pale yellow powder - 6% Na_2CO_3 and nitrogen to prevent formation of free acid with CO_2	- 0.2% solution - 35% v/v Propylene glycol	- Only one chiral centre - Racemic mixture - S (+) enantiomer is 3–4 times more potent

(Continued)

	Propofol	Thiopental	Etomidate	Ketamine
Mechanism of action	- Enhancing γ-aminobutyric acid (GABA)-induced chloride current by binding to β subunit - Inhibition of NMDA receptors	- Enhances the action of GABA by increasing chloride conductance - Inhibition of NMDA receptors	- GABA receptor facilitation	- Non-competitive inhibition of NMDA receptors - Inhibits nor-adrenaline uptake
Pharmacodynamic effects	CVS: ↓HR, ↓SVR and ↓contractility Respiration: ↓ RR, suppression of laryngeal reflexes CNS: ↓ICP, ↓CBF and dystonic choreiform movements Gut: Anti-emetic effect by antagonism of dopamine D2 receptor Urine: Turns green Injection: Pain on injection	CVS: ↑HR, ↓SVR and ↓contractility Respiration: ↓ RR, broncho-spasm and laryngo-spasm CNS: ↓ICP, ↓CBF and ↓CMRO$_2$ Renal: Urine retention due to ↑ADH (morphine has similar action)	CVS: ↓SVR but HR, BP and contractility unchanged (cardio stable) Respiration: ↓ RR CNS: ↓ICP, ↓CBF, myoclonus Endocrine: ↓ Cortisol formation by inhibiting 11β-hydroxy-lase and 17α-hydroxy-lase Injection: Pain on injection	CVS: ↑HR, ↑BP, ↑ cardiac output and no change in SVR - Direct cardiac depressant effect Respiration: ↑ RR, Preserved laryngeal reflexes, Bronchodilation CNS: ↑ ICP and ↑CBF. Dissociative anaesthesia Gut: Causes nausea and vomiting. Salivation Pain: Analgesia along with sedation
pH	7	10.8	8.1	3.5–5.5
pKa	11	7.6	4.1	7.5
Protein binding (%)	98	80	75	25

(*Continued*)

	Propofol	Thiopental	Etomidate	Ketamine
Volume of distribution (L/kg)	4	2.5	3	3
Clearance (mL/kg/min)	30–60	3.5	10–20	17
Elimination half-life (h)	5–12	6–15	1–4	2
Metabolism	- Metabolised by **glucuronidation at position 1** and hydroxylation in liver - Metabolism in lungs as well	- Metabolism by hepatic oxidation - Active metabolite is pentobarbitone	- Metabolised by plasma and **hepatic esterases**	- *N-demethylation and hydroxylation in liver* - Norketamine is active metabolite
Side effects	- Propofol infusion syndrome in doses greater than 4 mg/kg/hr (heart failure, rhabdomyolysis, acidosis) - Epileptiform movements	- Anaphylaxis 1 in 20,000 - Thrombosis if intra-arterial - ANT antianalgesia - **Porphyrinogen**	- Nausea and vomiting - Antiplatelet - Porphyrinogen	- Nausea and vomiting - Emergence delirium - **Porphyrinogen**
Doses	- Induction dose: 1–2.5 mg/kg - Maintenance of GA: 50–150 µg/kg/min - Sedation: 25–75 µg/kg/min - Antiemetic action: 10–20 mg iv	Induction dose: 3–4 mg/kg	- Induction dose: **0.2–0.3 mg/kg**	- Induction dose: 0.5–2 mg/kg IV or 4–6 mg/kg IM - Sedation and analgesia: 0.2–0.8 mg/kg IV or 2–4 mg/kg IM - Preventive analgesia: 0.15–0.25 mg/kg IV

Opioids

- Basic amines
- **Opiate:** Naturally occurring compounds that are derived from opium
  - **Opioid:** Synthetic substance that acts on the opioid receptor
- **Natural compounds:** Morphine, codeine
  - **Semi-synthetic compounds:** Diamorphine, buprenorphine, oxycodone
  - **Synthetic compounds:** Pethidine, fentanyl, alfentanil, remifentanil, methadone
- **Mechanism of action:** *G-protein-coupled receptors:* $G_i \rightarrow \downarrow$ cAMP $\rightarrow \downarrow$ neurotransmitter
  - **Blocks voltage gated Ca^{2+} channels**
  - *Hyperpolarisation by K efflux*
- **Classification of opioid receptors**

Receptor	Location	Effects
MOP, mu, μ	Brain, spinal cord	Analgesia, physical dependence Respiratory depression, CVS depression Euphoria, miosis, constipation
KOP, kappa, K	Brain	Analgesia, Dysphoria (No respiratory depression)
DOP, delta, δ	Brain, spinal cord	Analgesia, physical dependence Respiratory depression
NOP	Brain, spinal cord	Anxiety, depression

- **Pharmacodynamic effects**
  - **Analgesia:** Visceral pain
  - **Respiratory depression:** Sensitivity of brainstem to CO_2 is reduced following opioid
  - **CVS:** Mild bradycardia and hypotension due to histamine release, vagal stimulation, sympatholysis
  - **CNS:** Sedation and euphoria
  - **Gastrointestinal tract (GIT):** Constricts all the sphincters of gut
  - **Urinary:** Urinary retention
  - **Nausea and vomiting:** Chemoreceptor trigger zone (CTZ) is stimulated via 5-HT$_3$ and dopamine receptors
  - **Pruritus:** Not due to histamine release

- o **Muscle rigidity:** Large doses can cause muscle rigidity
- o **Miosis:** Stimulation of Edinger–Westphal nucleus
- o **Endocrine:** Antidiuretic hormone (ADH) secretion is increased
- **Morphine:** Metabolised in liver and kidney to morphine 3-glucuronide (60%) and morphine 6-glucuronide (10%). **Morphine 6-glucuronide is 13 times more potent than morphine and accumulates in renal failure**
- **Diamorphine:** Diamorphine is a **synthetic deacetylated morphine** with *no affinity for opioid receptor.* It produces the greatest degree of euphoria among opioids
- **Pethidine:** Used during labour. Longer half-life and more lipid soluble than morphine. Metabolism produces norpethidine, which accumulates in fetus peaking 4 hours after maternal intramuscular dose. Norpethidine accumulates after renal failure as well. Norpethidine can cause hallucinations and seizures. Dose is 0.5–1 mg/kg
  - o Chemically related to atropine and has some atropine-like effects along with some local anaesthetic activity
  - o **Protein binding: 65–75%**
  - o Out of all the opioids, pethidine shifts the log dose response the most to the right because of highest doses used (75 mg)

Parameters	Morphine	Diamorphine	Fentanyl	Alfentanil	Remifentanil
Relative lipid solubility	1	250 (Subcutaneous)	600	90	20
Relative potency	1	2	100	10–20	100
pKa	8.0	7.6	8.4	6.5	7.1
Protein binding (%)	35	40	83	90 (highest)	70
Oral bioavailability (%)	25-30	Low	33	N/A	N/A
Volume of distribution (L/kg)	3.5	5	4	0.6	0.3
Clearance mL/kg/min	16	3.1	13	6	40
Elimination rate (min)	170	5	190	100	10

(Continued)

Parameters	Morphine	Diamorphine	Fentanyl	Alfentanil	Remifentanil
Metabolism	Glucuroni-dation and N-demeth-ylation	Ester hydroly-sis to monoacetyl-morphine	N-Deal-kylation, then hydrox-ylation	N-demeth-ylation	Plasma and tissue esterases
Dose	100–200 µg/kg	75–100 µg/kg	1–2 µg/kg	5–25 µg/kg	0.05–2 µg/kg/min

- Fentanyl: High therapeutic index of 400
- Equivalent doses of opioids

Drug	Route	Dose
Morphine	IV	5 mg
Morphine	Oral	10 mg
Diamorphine	IV	3 mg
Codeine	Oral	100 mg
Tramadol	Oral	100 mg
Oxycodone	Oral	6.6
Fentanyl	Transdermal	Fentanyl 25 µg/hr = oral morphine 60 mg/24 hr
Buprenorphine	Transdermal	Buprenorphine 5 µg/hr = oral morphine 12 mg/24 hr

- Alfentanil: 90% un-ionized at pH 7.4
- Tramadol: Agonist actions at all opioid receptors, but particularly at µ-receptors. It also inhibits reuptake of noradrenaline and 5-HT. Produces less respiratory depression and constipation than, morphine. Can precipitate *seizures*. Can interact with selective serotonin reuptake inhibitors (SSRIs)/ monoamine oxidase (MAO) inhibitors to cause serotonin syndrome
- Methadone: High oral bioavailability of 75% and long acting. Used for weaning heroin addicts. Less sedative than morphine
- Buprenorphine: Partial agonist. Long duration of action. Analgesia at low concentrations by µ-receptor stimulation. Increasing doses influence the nociception opioid peptide (NOP) receptor, which is anti-analgesic
- Codeine phosphate: *Contraindicated in children under the age of 12 years*
- Naloxone: Pure opioid antagonist. Can cause hypertension and pulmonary oedema. Dose is 1–4 µg/kg. Duration of action is 30–40 min, so infusion may be required

Non-steroidal anti-inflammatory drugs

- **Mechanism of action:** Phospholipase A_2 acts on cell phospholipid bilayer to produce arachidonic acid
  - Cyclooxygenase (COX) acts on arachidonic acid to produce thromboxane, prostacyclin and prostaglandins. Non-steroidal anti-inflammatory drugs (NSAIDs) block this pathway
  - Lipoxygenase also acts on arachidonic acid to produce leukotrienes. Arachidonic acid leftover after COX being blocked enters this pathway and produces **leukotrienes, which cause NSAID-induced asthma**
- **COX**
  - **COX-1:** Constitutive form that is found in most cells and is responsible for maintaining renal blood flow and gastric mucus production. Production of thromboxane
  - **COX-2:** Inducible form that is found in macrophages when tissue damage occurs. COX-2 helps in production of prostacyclin 2
  - **COX-3:** CNS variant of COX-1. Paracetamol acts on it
- **Classification of NSAIDs**
  - **Non-specific COX inhibitors:** Aspirin, diclofenac, paracetamol, ibuprofen, ketorolac
  - **Specific COX-2 inhibitors:** Parecoxib, etoricoxib
- **Function of arachidonic acid products**
  - PGE_2: ↓Gastric acid, ↑ gastric mucus production
    - **Dinoprostone** is a naturally occurring prostaglandin E_1 used for labour induction, bleeding after delivery, termination of pregnancy, and in newborn babies to keep the ductus arteriosus open
  - PGE_1: Relaxes vascular smooth muscle
    - **Alprostadil** is a synthetic analogue of PGE_1 used to maintain patency of ductus arteriosus in neonates and erectile dysfunction in adults
    - **Misoprostol** is another analogue of PGE_1 used to reduce the risk of NSAID-related ulcers, prevent postpartum haemorrhage (PPH) and for first trimester abortions
  - $PGF_{2\alpha}$: Uterine contraction and bronchoconstriction
    - **Carboprost** is synthetic analogue of $PGF_{2\alpha}$ used for PPH
    - **Latanoprost** is a synthetic analogue of $PGF_{2\alpha}$ used to treat elevated intraocular pressure (IOP)
  - **PGI_2 (Prostacyclin):** Vasodilator
    - **Epoprostenol:** Synthetic prostacyclin analogue used in pulmonary artery hypertension
  - **Thromboxane:** Vasoconstrictor and platelet aggregator

- **Side effects of NSAIDs**
  - ○ **Gastric ulceration:** Ketorolac and piroxicam have the highest risk. Ibuprofen (<1.2 g/day) has the lowest risk factors amongst non-selective COX inhibitors. COX-2 inhibitors have lower risk than non-selective ones
  - ○ **Vascular events: Myocardial infarction in COX-2 inhibitors**
  - ○ **Renal toxicity:** Prolonged use can cause papillary necrosis and inter-stitial fibrosis
  - ○ **Hepatotoxicity:** Rise in serum transaminase levels even following short-term intake
  - ○ **Asthma:** Due to uninhibited leukotriene pathway
  - ○ **Drug interactions:** Heparin or warfarin may be displaced from its protein binding sites

Chemical	Aspirin	Paracetamol
Mechanism of action	- Low-dose **irreversible** blockade of COX-1 and, hence, thromboxane - High dose blocks COX-2 as well	Central blockade of COX-3
Pharmaco-dynamics/ Side effects	- CVS: Cardioprotective at low dose due to blockage of thromboxane - Respiration: Asthma - GI: Gastric ulcer and liver dysfunction	- CNS: Analgesia and antipyretic - Rapid injection can cause hypotension - Overdose can cause acute liver failure - Idiopathic thrombocytopenia - Analgesic nephropathy
Pharmaco-kinetics	- Absorbed mainly in small intestine as pKa of 3.5 - Plasma protein binding: 85% - Hepatic and intestinal metabo-lism by **esterases** to salicylic acid - First-order kinetic in low dose, zero order in overdose - Aspirin inhibits renal secretion of urate and not urea	- Hepatic metabolism to glucuronide and sulphate metabolites - 10% metabolism to N-acetyl-p-amino benzoquinoneimine (NAPQI), which is toxic - Plasma protein binding: 10% - **Used as a marker of testing gastric emptying**
Uses and dose	- Angina and stroke prophylaxis: 75 mg OD - Post-MI and thrombotic stroke: 300 mg one off f/b 75 mg OD - Analgesia: 300–900 mg 6 hourly	- Fever: 10–15mg/kg 6 hourly - Analgesia: 15–20 mg/kg 6 hourly

Chemical	Diclofenac	Ibuprofen
Mechanism of action	Inhibits COX-1 and -2 equally	Inhibits COX-1 and -2 equally
Pharmaco-dynamics/ Side effects	- CVS: Reversible inhibition of platelet function, risk of coronary events similar to COX-2 inhibitors - Less GI upset than aspirin - Asthma	- CVS: Dose <1.2 g/day is not prothrombotic - Weak anti-inflammatory effect at dose of <1.2 g/day but lesser side effects compared with other NSAIDs as well
Pharmaco-kinetics	- Oral bioavailability: 60% - Plasma protein binding: 99.5%	- Oral bioavailability: 80% - Plasma protein binding: 99%
Uses	Analgesia: 1 mg/kg 8 hourly	Analgesia: 10 mg/kg tds

Chemical	Ketorolac	Parecoxib
Mechanism of action	Inhibits COX-1 and -2 equally	- Selective COX-2 inhibitor - Prodrug converted to valdecoxib, which blocks COX-2
Pharmaco-dynamics/ Side effects	- Potent analgesic effect but weak anti-inflammatory effect - Potent anti-pyretic as well - Maximum GI toxicity when taken orally	- No action of its own - Valdecoxib has been withdrawn due to serious dermatological side effects - Parecoxib still used because of its short-term use as just a perioperative pain analgesic
Pharmaco-kinetics	- Oral bioavailability: 85% - Plasma protein binding: 99%	Plasma protein binding: 98%
Uses	- Analgesia: IV 10–30 mg 6 hourly - Maximum: 90 mg in non-elderly and 60 mg in elderly	Perioperative pain: 40 mg IV dose f/b 20–40 mg 6–12 hourly to a maximum of 80 mg/day

- NSAIDs: Weak acids, small volume of distribution (0.1–0.2 L/kg) and high protein binding (99%)
  - Even intravenous (IV) injection will cause gastric mucosal damage
- Sumatriptan: Used in treatment of migraine and cluster headaches. Can cross BBB
  - 5-HT$_1$ agonist. Can cause both tachycardia and bradycardia
- Paracetamol: In a healthy individual, giving twice the dose of paracetamol won't hurt and safe daily dose of paracetamol of 4 g/day shouldn't be exceeded. However, it can cause toxicity relatively easily because the hepatic enzyme pathways are easily saturated in overdose

Suxamethonium

- Two molecules of acetylcholine are bound by acetyl group
- Stored at 4°C. Elimination half-life of 4–5 min
- 10 Genotypes, 4 Alleles, including silent (Es), usual (Eu), atypical (Ea) and fluoride resistant (Ef)
- **Most prolonged duration:** Homozygous silent, homozygous atypical, heterozygous silent atypical
- **Dibucaine:** Inhibits normal plasma cholinesterase. Variant forms are not blocked
- **Eu:** Eu is 80 (Incidence 96% of population), Ea:Ea is 20 (Incidence, 1:29,000)
- **Acquired causes of suxamethonium apnoea** are mostly no longer than 30 min and **causes are**
  - Pregnancy
  - Renal failure
  - Cardiac failure
  - Liver failure
  - Hyperthyroidism
  - Cancer
  - Lithium
  - Oral contraceptive pills (OCPs)
  - Metoclopramide
  - Ester local anaesthetics
- **Produces dual block:** Phase 2 block due to presynaptic effect
- **Side effects:** Hyperkalaemia (>10% burns patients), **Bradycardia (repeated doses),** muscle pain (young females)
- Intramuscular (IM) injection can be given but painful
- **Anaphylaxis rate of 11.1/100,000 administrations is greater compared with 5.88/100,000 of that of rocuronium**
- Metabolised by plasma or pseudocholinesterase to succinylmonocholine which is metabolised to succinic acid and choline
- Very little excreted in urine (10%)
- **Nodal bradycardia:** Direct nodal muscarinic receptor stimulation
- Increases IOP by 10 mm Hg, intragastric pressure by 10 cm H_2O

- Confusion busting vignette
  - o **Red cell esterase:** Esmolol
  - o **Hepatic and intestinal esterase:** Aspirin
  - o **Plasma cholinesterase:** Suxamethonium, mivacurium, procaine and tetracaine (ester group of local anaesthetics [LAs])
  - o **Non-specific plasma esterases:** Atracurium
  - o **Non-specific plasma and tissue esterase:** Remifentanil
  - o **Non-specific liver esterase:** Etomidate
  - o Diamorphine is also metabolised by esterases

Non-depolarising muscle relaxants

	Aminosteroids			Benzylisoquinoliniums		
	Ro-curonium	Ve-curonium	Pan-curonium	Atracurium	Cis-atracurium	Mivacurium
Structure	Monoquaternary		Bisquater-nary	10 stereoiso-mers	One of the 10 stereoiso-mers of atracurium	3 stereoisomers
Intubation dose (mg/kg)	0.6 0.9 (rapid sequence induction [RSI])	0.1	0.1	0.5	0.2	0.2
Speed of onset	Rapid	Medium				
Duration	Medium		Long	Medium		Short
Protein binding (%)	10	10	20–60	15	15	10
Volume of distribu-tion (L/kg)	0.2	0.2	0.3	0.15	0.15	0.2–0.3
Metabolism (%)	20	<5	30	90	95	90
Elimination in bile (%)	70	60	20	0	0	0
Elimination in urine (%)	30	40	80	10	5	5

(Continued)

	Aminosteroids			Benzylisoquinoliniums		
	Ro-curonium	Ve-curonium	Pan-curonium	Atracurium	Cis-atracurium	Mivacurium
Cardiovascular effects	None/↓ HR	None	↑ HR	None		
Histamine release	Rare			Slight	Rare	Slight
Renal failure	Prolonged effect			No effect		
Notes	- Unstable in solution - 3 active metabolites, accumulation with repeated dosing	- Rapid onset vecuronium	- Vagolytic - One active 3-hydroxy metabolite	- Hofmann elimination is spontaneous degradation of a quaternary ammonium to a tertiary amine (laudanosine) - Is epileptogenic	- Less histamine release - Longer onset of action, **four times more potent** and longer duration than atracurium - Hofmann degradation	- Mixture of 3 stereoisomers - Trans-trans, cis-trans, cis-cis

- Competitive neuromuscular blockade increased by
  - Hypothermia
  - Metabolic acidosis
  - Hypokalaemia
  - Hypocalcaemia
  - Lithium
  - Calcium channel blockers
  - Aminoglycosides
- Competitive neuromuscular blockade decreased by
  - Acetylcholinesterase inhibitor like edrophonium
  - Hepatic enzyme inducers like phenytoin and carbamazepine

Mivacurium with plasma cholinesterase deficiency can prolong the neuromuscular block to 2 hours with two twitches on train of four (TOF).

A drug that is more potent than rocuronium will be given at a smaller dose; therefore, it takes longer to work.

Neuromuscular reversal agents

- Neuromuscular reversal agents can be divided into anticholinesterases and γ-cyclodextrins
- Anticholinesterases inhibit the action of enzyme acetylcholinesterase and prevent breakdown of acetylcholine. They can be classified as
  - Short acting: Edrophonium. Competitive antagonism. Duration 10–20 min
    - *Edrophonium:* Used for diagnosis of myasthenia gravis or to exclude cholinergic crisis
  - Intermediate acting: Neostigmine, pyridostigmine, physostigmine
    - *Pyridostigmine:* Treatment of myasthenia gravis
    - *Physostigmine:* Treatment of glaucoma
  - Long acting: Echothiophate. Phosphorylation of enzyme
    - *Echothiophate:* Treatment of glaucoma

	Neostigmine	Sugammadex
Chemical	Anticholinesterase (AChE) **quaternary amine**	γ-Cyclodextrin
Mechanism of action	- **Carbamylate** is the ester site of AChE and blocks it - This increases acetylcholine at neuromuscular junction (NMJ) allowing reversal of neuromuscular block	- Ring-like structure encapsulates drug in lipophilic core and separates it from NMJ - Effective only for rocuronium and **vecuronium** reversal
Effects	- CVS: Bradycardia and hypotension - Respiration: Bronchoconstriction and increased secretions - CNS: Miosis and blurred vision - GIT: Nausea and vomiting, peristalsis, increased secretions - Used along with glycopyrrolate to counter side effects	- CVS: Stable - **Post-sugammadex dose, wait for 24 hours before readministering rocuronium/vecuronium** - Avoid if creatinine clearance <30 mL/min
Pharmacokinetics	- **Oral bioavailability: 1–2%** - Protein binding: 10% - V_D: 0.4–1 L/kg - Effect in 10 mins and lasts 4 hours - Shorter acting than pyridostigmine	- Only given intravenously - No protein binding - Excreted from kidneys unchanged with $T_{1/2}$ of 2.5 hr

(Continued)

	Neostigmine	Sugammadex
Uses	- Reversal of neuromuscular blockade - Paralytic ileus in absence of true mechanical obstruction - Myasthenia gravis	- Routine reversal of neuromuscular blockade - Emergency reversal due to failed intubation after rapid sequence induction (RSI)
Dose	- 0.05 mg/kg	- Immediate emergency reversal due to failed intubation: 16 mg/kg - Post-tetanic count 1 or 2: 4 mg/kg - 2 Twitches on TOF: 2 mg/kg

Local anaesthetics

- **Mechanism of action:** Blockade of Na^+ channel. Un-ionised drug enters the cell through phospholipid membranes. It becomes ionised in axoplasm and blocks the Na^+ channel in its inactivated state
- **Classification:** Esters and amides. Linkage between lipophilic aromatic group and hydrophilic amine chain
  - Esters: For example, cocaine, **tetracaine (amethocaine)**, procaine. Hydrolysis by pseudocholinesterase in plasma. **Fast terminal elimination time**
    - Unstable in solution
    - Hypersensitivity reactions due to metabolic product p-aminobenzoic acid
  - **Amides:** Lignocaine, bupivacaine, ropivacaine, **prilocaine**. Metabolism by amidases in liver. Crosses placenta as lipid soluble
    - Shelf life of 2 years
    - Bound to α-1 acid glycoprotein with high affinity
- **Physiochemical properties:** Weak bases
  - **Potency:** Greater the lipid solubility, more is the potency
  - **Speed of onset:** Molecules with pKa closer to pH 7.4 will be more un-ionised and faster acting. *Dose increase will fasten as more drug available for action*
  - **Duration of action:** Higher the protein binding, longer is the action
  - **Vasodilation:** Prilocaine (maximum) > lidocaine > bupivacaine > ropivacaine
  - **Systemic absorption sites:** Intercostal (maximum) > caudal > epidural > brachial plexus > subcutaneous

Drug	Onset of action	pKa	Plasma protein binding (%)	Elimination half-life (min)	Maximum dose
Cocaine	Moderate	8.6	95	80	3 mg/kg
Amethocaine	Slow	8.5	75	100	1.5 mg/kg
Lidocaine	Fast	7.9	70	100	3 mg/kg 7 mg /kg (adrenaline)
Prilocaine	Fast	7.7	55	100	6 mg/kg 8 mg/kg (felypressin)
Ropivacaine	Moderate	8.1	94	120	3 mg/kg
Bupivacaine	Moderate	8.1	95	160	2 mg/kg

- Eutectic mixture of local anaesthetic (EMLA)
  - 2.5% Lidocaine and 2.5% prilocaine
  - Methaemoglobinaemia is caused by ortho-Toluidine, a metabolite of prilocaine
- Intravenous regional anaesthesia (IVRA): Use less cardiotoxic drug like *prilocaine 5 mg/kg*
- Toxic dose of lidocaine is >5 μg/mL compared with 1.5 μg/mL of bupivacaine
- Levobupivacaine is the S-enantiomer of bupivacaine. It is less cardiotoxic
- Ropivacaine: Motor block produced is slower in onset, less dense and of shorter duration
  - Ropivacaine has more lipid solubility and is four times more potent than lidocaine
- Intralipid: Lipid emulsion used in Local anaesthetic systemic toxicity (circumoral tingling, seizures, arrhythmias and cardiac arrest)
  - Dose: 1.5 mg/kg bolus followed by infusion at 0.25 mL/kg/min. Two more boluses at 5-min intervals (total 3 boluses). Increase infusion rate to 0.5 mL/kg/min

Systemic Pharmacology

12

Antihypertensive drugs

Classification of antihypertensive drugs

- Heart
  - Beta-blockers
- Blood vessels
  - Directly acting vasodilators
    - **Sodium nitroprusside:** Both arterial and venous dilator
    - **Glyceryl trinitrate:** Venous dilator
  - Indirectly acting vasodilators
    - **Alpha blockers:** Doxazosin, prazosin, phenoxybenzamine, phentolamine
    - **Calcium channel blockers:** Amlodipine, nimodipine, nifedipine
    - **Potassium channel blockers:** Nicorandil
    - Magnesium
- Kidneys
  - **Diuretics:** Frusemide
  - **Agents acting on renin-angiotensin-aldosterone system:** Enalapril, losartan
- Central nervous system (CNS)
  - **Centrally acting drugs:** Clonidine, methyldopa
  - **Ganglion blockers:** Trimetaphan

	Glyceryl trinitrate	Sodium nitroprusside
Mechanism of action	GTN → NO → cGMP → vasodilation	SNP → NO → cGMP →vasodilation
Pharmacodynamics/ Side effects	- CVS: ↓ SVR mainly by venodilation, ↑ HR - CNS: ↑ ICP leading to headache - Tolerance to patches but not to infusions, so patch free period every day	- CVS: ↓ SVR by both arteriolar and venodilation, ↑ HR - CNS: ↑ ICP leading to headache - Respiratory: ↓ Hypoxic pulmonic vasoconstriction

(Continued)

DOI: 10.1201/9781003390244-14

	Glyceryl trinitrate	Sodium nitroprusside
Mechanism of action	- Methaemoglobin rarely	- Tachyphylaxis - Toxicity: CN^- Levels >8 µg/mL, CN^- + cytochrome c → lactic acidosis, Cyanokit (hydroxyco-balamin) for treatment
Pharmaco-kinetics	- Well absorbed sublingually but **oral bioavailability is less than 5%**	-> SNP + haemoglobin → NO + $5CN^-$ + methaemoglobin -> $1CN^-$ + methaemoglobin → cyanomethaemoglobin -> $4CN^-$ + thiosulphate → thiocyanate
Indications of use	- Pulmonary oedema (infusion) - Treatment and prophylaxis of angina (tablet, patch, spray) - Uncontrolled hypertension (infusion) - Anal fissures (ointment)	- Uncontrolled hypertension
Dose	- Severe LVF: 20–25 µg/min until 200 µg/min	- Uncontrolled hypertension: 0.5–6 µg/kg/min

	Phenoxybenzamine	Phentolamine
Mechanism of action	Long-acting irreversible non-selective α_1 blocker	Competitive non-selective α_1 blocker
Pharmaco-dynamics/ Side effects	- CVS: ↓ SVR, ↑ HR - CNS: Sedation, miosis - Impotence, contact dermatitis	- CVS: ↓ SVR, ↑ HR - Respiratory: Bronchospasm due to presence of sulphites - Increases insulin release leading to hypoglycaemia
Pharmaco-kinetics	- Oral bioavailability: 25% - Effect persists for 3 days as new receptors are synthesised	- Oral bioavailability: 20% but not used orally - Elimination half-life is 20 min
Indications of use	- Preoperative control of BP in patients of phaeochromocy-toma	- Preoperative control of BP in patients of phaeochromocytoma - Chronic pain - Erectile dysfunction

(*Continued*)

	Phenoxybenzamine	Phentolamine
Dose	- 10 mg orally titrated to max of 1–2 mg/kg in two divided doses - IV dose is via central cannula, in dose of 1 mg/kg	- Preoperative control of BP in patients of phaeochromocytoma: 1–5 mg IV bolus followed by 6–40 mg/hr

	Nimodipine	Nifedipine
Mechanism of action	- Dihydropyridine calcium channel antagonist	- Dihydropyridine calcium channel antagonist
Pharmaco-dynamics/ Side effects	- CVS: ↓ SVR, ↑ HR, arteriolar dilatation but ↓ contractility - CNS: Headache, vertigo	- CVS: ↓ SVR, ↑ HR, arteriolar dilatation but ↓ contractility - Oedema of legs - CNS: Headache, vertigo
Pharmaco-kinetics	- Oral bioavailability: 28% - Protein binding: 98%	- Oral bioavailability: 65%, sublingual route avoids first-pass metabolism - Protein binding: 95% - $t_{1/2}$: 5 hours
Indications of use	- Reduction of vasospasm in subarachnoid haemorrhage (SAH) - Migraine	- Hypertension (can be given with α antagonists) - Raynaud's phenomenon - Angina
Dose	- Oral: 60 mg 4 hourly - IV: 1–2 mg/hr	- 10–20 mg 8 hourly

	Ramipril	Losartan
Mechanism of action	- Prodrug: Converted to ramiprilat - Competitive ACE inhibitor	- Angiotensin II receptors blockers (ARBs)
Pharmaco-dynamics/ Side effects	- CVS: ↓ SVR, ↑ HR - Renal: ↓ Aldosterone → ↑ K^+, contraindicated in bilateral renal artery stenosis - **Cough**, angioedema, agranulocytosis	- CVS: ↓ SVR, ↑ HR, first dose hypotension - **No cough like that with ramipril** - Contraindicated in bilateral renal artery stenosis

(Continued)

	Ramipril	Losartan
	- If cough becomes a problem, replace it with ARBs	- Refractory hypotension perioperatively (omit 24 hours before surgery)
Pharmaco-kinetics	- Oral bioavailability: 50% - Converted to ramiprilat by liver esterases - $t_{1/2}$: 15 hours	- Oral bioavailability: 30% - Protein binding: 99% - Elimination $t_{1/2}$: 2 hours and that of active metabolite is 7 hours
Indications of use	- Hypertension - Heart failure - Myocardial infarction with left ventricular dysfunction	- Hypertension
Dose	- Oral: 1.25 mg–10 mg	- 25–50 mg

	Clonidine	Dexmedetomidine
Mechanism of action	- α_2 agonist. α_2: α_1:: 200:1	- α_2 agonist. α_2: α_1:: 1600:1
Pharmaco-dynamics/ Side effects	- CVS: ↓ SVR, ↓ HR - CNS: Sedation, ↓ 50% of MAC of volatile agents, analgesia - Renal: ↓ ADH → diuresis	- CVS: ↓ SVR, ↓ HR, May cause first- or second-degree block - CNS: Sedation, ↓ 50% of MAC of volatile agents, analgesia - Respiratory depression
Pharmaco-kinetics	- Oral bioavailability: 100% - Protein binding: 20% - Elimination half-life: 9–18 hours - Dose reduced in renal impairment	- Distribution half-life of approximately 6 min - Protein binding: 94% - Elimination half-life: 2–4 hours
Indications of use	- Hypertension - Acute and chronic pain - Opioid withdrawal - Sedation in mechanically ventilated patients	- Sedation during intensive care - Adjunct in general anaesthesia
Dose	- Oral: 50–600 µg 8 hourly - IV: 75–300 µg 8 hourly	- Sedation: 0.7 µg/kg/hr followed by 0.2–1.4 µg/kg/hr

Clonidine inhibits ADH but morphine and thiopentone cause secretion of antidiuretic hormone (ADH).

	Methyldopa	Hydralazine
Mechanism of action	- Metabolised to α-methyl noradrenaline which is an α₂ agonist	- Dihydropyridine calcium channel antagonist
Pharmaco-dynamics/ side effects	- CVS: ↓ SVR, ↓ HR - CNS: Sedation, MAC of volatile agents is reduced - Positive direct Coombs test in 10–20% patients - Autoimmune haemolytic anaemia - Liver dysfunction	- CVS: ↓ SVR, ↑ HR, oedema - CNS: Headache - Renal: ↓ Urine output - Peripheral neuropathy and blood dyscrasias - Lupus erythematosus type syndrome
Pharmaco-kinetics	- Oral bioavailability: 10–60% - Protein binding: 50%	- Oral bioavailability: 25–55% depending on **acetylator status** - Protein binding: 90% - $t_{1/2}$: 2–3 hours
Indications of use	- Pregnancy-induced hypertension and pre-eclampsia	- Chronic hypertension - Pregnancy-induced hypertension - CHF
Dose	- 0.5–3 g/day in 2–3 doses orally	- Hypertension: 25–50 mg 12 hourly orally - Pregnancy: 5–10 mg IV every 20–30 min - CHF: 25 mg 6 hourly, 50 mg 6 hourly orally

	Doxazocin	Nicorandil
Mechanism of action	- Highly selective α₁ antagonist	- Activates K⁺ channels open → K⁺ moves out of cell → hyperpolarisation → ↓ Ca²⁺ → ↓ cardiac work
Pharmaco-dynamics/ side effects	- CVS: ↓ SVR, no reflex tachycardia, postural hypotension - CNS: Headache, vertigo - Impotence and priapism	- CVS: ↓ preload, ↓ cardiac work - CNS: Headache, vertigo - Angio-oedema
Pharmaco-kinetics	- Oral bioavailability: 60–70% - Protein binding: 98% - Elimination $t_{1/2}$: 9–12 hours	- Oral bioavailability: 75% - Protein binding: 0% - $t_{1/2}$: 1 hour
Indications of use	- Hypertension - Benign prostate hypertrophy	- Angina: Treatment and prophylaxis
Dose	Hypertension: Oral: 1 mg daily to max of 16 mg/day	- 10–30 mg 12 hourly orally

Antiarrhythmic drugs

- Vaughn–Williams classification of antiarrhythmic drugs

Class	Mechanism	Drugs	Action Potential
Ia	Sodium channel blockade	Quinidine Procainamide Disopyramide	- Prolongs action potential and refractory period
Ib		Lignocaine Phenytoin Mexiletine	- Shortens action potential and refractory period
Ic		Flecainide Propafenone	- No effect
II	Beta-blockers	Esmolol Propranolol Atenolol	- Slows rate at SA node and reduces AV conduction - Prolongs action potential and refractory period
III	K+ channel blockers	Amiodarone Sotalol Bretylium	- Slows rate at SA node and reduces AV conduction - Prolongs action potential and refractory period
IV	Ca^{2+} channel blockers	Verapamil Diltiazem	- Slows rate at SA node and reduces AV conduction - Prolongs action potential and refractory period

- Classification based on clinical use

Arrhythmias	Drugs
SVT	Adenosine, verapamil, diltiazem, beta-blockers, digoxin, quinidine
VT	Lignocaine, mexiletine
SVT and VT	Amiodarone, sotalol, flecainide, propafenone, procainamide, disopyramide
Digoxin toxicity	Phenytoin

Drugs	Quinidine Ia	Lignocaine Ib	Flecainide Ic
Chemical	- Enantiomer of quinine - Bark of the cin-chona tree	Amide local anaesthetic	Amide local anaesthetic
Mechanism of action	- Blocks fast Na^+ channels - ↓ Vagal tone	- Blocks fast Na^+ channels - ↓ Vagal tone	- Blocks fast Na^+ channels
Pharmaco-dynamics/ Side effects	- CVS: ↑ QRS, ↑ QT interval, hypoten-sion, torsades de pointes - CNS: Cinchonism, i.e., tinnitus, blurred vision, hearing loss, headache, confusion - Diarrhoea - Thrombocytopenia	Signs of toxicity >4 µg/mL: Perioral tingling, tinnitus >5 µg/mL: Coma, seizures >10 µg/mL: Cardiac arrest	- CVS: May precipi-tate pre-existing conduction disorders - May precipitate heart failure - CNS: Dizziness, paraesthesia, headaches
Pharmacoki-netics	- Metabolised by cytochrome P450 in liver - Oral bioavailability: 75% - Protein binding: ~90%	- Metabolised by amidases in liver - Given IV only for arrhythmias	- Metabolised by amidases in liver - Can be given orally, 90% bioavailability - Protein binding: ~50%
Uses	- Termination of SVTs including AF/flutter	- Sustained ven-tricular tachyar-rhythmias	- Termination of AF, VT and WPW
Dose	- AF: 300–400 mg PO q6h - PSVT: 400–600 mg PO q2-3h until paroxysm termi-nated	- Bolus 1 mg/kg fol-lowed by 1–3 mg/min	- Oral: 100 mg BD (maximum 400 mg) - IV: 2 mg/kg over 30 min followed by 1.5 mg/kg/hr and then 100–250 µg/kg/hr

Drugs	Amiodarone	Digoxin	Adenosine
Chemical	Iodinated benzofuran	Glycoside	Purine nucleoside
Mechanism of action	- Blocks K$^+$ channels - Class III antiarrhythmic but has properties of I, II and IV as well	- Inhibits Na$^+$/K$^+$ ATPase pump → ↑ Intracellular Na$^+$ → Inhibits Na$^+$/Ca^{2+} ATPase pump → ↑ Intracellular Ca^{2+} - ↑ Vagal tone	- Adenosine A1 receptor leads to hyperpolarised membrane - ↓ cAMP-mediated catecholamines stimulation of ventricles
Pharmacodynamics	- CVS: Hypotension, Bradycardia, Prolonged QT - CNS: Corneal microdeposits, halos and blurred vision (reversible) - Respiratory: Pneumonitis (diffuse pulmonary alveolitis) - GI: Cirrhosis, jaundice, hepatitis - Skin: Slate grey skin, photosensitivity - Endocrine: Hypo/hyperthyroidism (reversible)	- CVS: Premature ventricular ectopics, bigeminy, AV blocks, long PR interval - CNS: Visual disturbances of red/green perception, headache, lethargy - GIT: Anorexia, diarrhoea, nausea and vomiting - Endocrine: Gynaecomastia	- CVS: Hypotension, bradycardia, C/I in WPW syndrome - CNS: Sense of impending doom - Respiratory: Chest discomfort, bronchospasm in asthmatics
Pharmacokinetics	- Bioavailability: 22–86% - Protein binding: 97% - T$_{1/2}$: 54 days - Metabolised by liver	- Bioavailability: 75% - Protein binding: 25% - T$_{1/2}$: 35 hours - 10% metabolised by liver, 60% excreted unchanged in urine - **Big loading dose as digoxin has high volume of distribution**	- Rapidly deaminated in plasma - T$_{1/2}$: 8–10 s

(*Continued*)

Drugs	Amiodarone	Digoxin	Adenosine
Uses	- Termination of SVT, VT and WPW like flecainide	- Slow ventricular rate in AF - Inotrope in heart failure	- To terminate re-entrant tachyarrhythmia (SVT)
Dose	- 300 mg IV (5 mg/kg) STAT followed by 900 mg (15 mg/kg/ day) IV over 24 hours - Oral: 200 mg TDS for 1 week, 200 mg BD for 1 week, 200 mg OD onwards	- Loading dose: 0.75–1.5 mg oral or 0.75 mg IV - Maintenance dose: 125–250 µg daily	- In large vein as fast bolus, 6 mg followed by 12 mg f/b 12 mg - Half the dose if in central venous access

Drugs	Verapamil	Diltiazem	Sotalol
Chemical	Papaverine calcium channel blocker	- Benzothiazepine - Calcium channel blocker	Beta-blocker
Mechanism of action	- Blocks L-type Ca^{2+} channels (mostly cardiac)	- Blocks L-type Ca^{2+} channels - (Cardiac and vessel smooth muscle)	- Blocks β_1 receptor on heart - Class I and III anti-arrhythmic activity
Pharmaco-dynamics/ Side effects	- CVS: ↓ HR, ↓ BP, CCF along with beta-blockers, contraindicated in WPW syndrome - CNS: Dizziness, headache - Potentiates effects of muscle relaxants - Local anaesthetic effect - Constipation	- CVS: ↓ HR, ↓ BP - C/I in WPW syndrome - Local anaes-thetic effect - Constipation	- CVS: ↓ HR, ↓ BP - Respiratory: Bronchospasm - Endocrine: Masking symptoms of hypoglycaemia
Pharmaco-kinetics	- Bioavailability: 20% - Protein binding: 90% - $T_{1/2}$: 5 hours	- Bioavailabil-ity: 35% - Protein binding: 80% - $T_{1/2}$: 5 hours	- Bioavailability: 90% - Not plasma protein bound and excreted un-changed in urine

(Continued)

Drugs	Verapamil	Diltiazem	Sotalol
Uses	- SVTs except WPW syndrome	- Prophylaxis and treatment of angina and hypertension - SVTs except WPW syndrome	- SVT - Ventricular premature beats - Spontaneous sustained VT 2° to cardiac ischaemia (better than lignocaine)
Dose	- 10 mg IV in SVT - 40–120 mg 8 hourly orally	- 20 mg IV in SVT - 60–120 mg 6–8 hourly orally	- 50–100 mg IV over 20 min - 80 mg daily in 1–2 divided doses increased to 160–320 mg daily

- **Disopyramide: Negative inotropy with no effect on blood vessels. This is its mechanism to lower blood pressure (BP)**
  - Used for treatment of ventricular extrasystoles as it causes all kinds of ventricular arrhythmias like VF, VT and torsades de pointes but doesn't cause ventricular extrasystole

Beta-blockers

- Competitive β adrenoreceptor antagonist
- **Pharmacodynamic effects/side effects**
  - **Cardiovascular (CVS):** ↓ BP, ↓ heart rate (HR), ↓ renin secretion by β_1 inhibition. Careful in heart failure
  - **Respiratory:** Bronchospasm, so careful in asthma/chronic obstructive pulmonary disease (COPD)
  - **CNS:** Crossing blood–brain barrier (BBB) can cause hallucinations, nightmares, depression, fatigue
  - **Metabolic:** ↑ Resting glucose, masks symptoms of hypoglycaemia, ↑ triglycerides
- **Uses:** Hypertension, angina, tachyarrhythmias, anxiety, glaucoma, migraine, hypertrophic obstructive cardiomyopathy (HOCM), phaeochromocytoma, obtund laryngoscopy response

- Beta-blockers with intrinsic sympathomimetic activity
  - Pindolol (max), acebutolol, labetalol, timolol (pneumonic for the drugs pindolol, acebutolol, labetalol, timolol [PALT])
- Beta-blockers' quinidine-like membrane stabilising effect
  - Propranolol (max), pindolol, acebutolol, labetalol, timolol (P-PALT)
- Non-selective beta-blocker
  - Propranolol, sotalol, timolol, labetalol ($\alpha + \beta$)
- β_1-selective blockers
  - Acebutolol, atenolol, bisoprolol, esmolol, metoprolol
- Atenolol: β_1-selective blocker. Dose is 50–100 mg orally, 2.5 mg intravenously (IV) slowly
  - Low lipid solubility, hence, excreted unchanged in urine without hepatic metabolism
  - *Oral bioavailability,* 45%; *protein bound,* 5%; *half-life,* 7 hours
- Esmolol: β_1-selective blocker. *Dose:* 50–300 µg/kg/min or 10 mg bolus IV
  - Metabolised by red blood cell esterases
  - *Protein bound,* 60%; *half-life,* 10 min
- Metoprolol: β_1-selective blocker. Dose is 50–200 mg orally, 5 mg IV slowly
  - *Oral bioavailability,* 50%; *protein bound,* 20%; *half-life,* 3–7 hours
- Bisoprolol: β_1-selective blocker. Dose is 1.25–10 mg orally
  - *Oral bioavailability,* 90%; *protein bound,* 30%; *half-life,* 10 hours
- Propranolol: Non-selective blocker. Dose is 160–320 mg orally, 0.5 mg IV up to 10 mg IV
  - Prevents the peripheral conversion of T4 → T3. Used in thyrotoxicosis
  - *Oral bioavailability,* 30%; *protein bound,* 90%; *half-life,* 4 hours
  - Can cause cold hands and feet due to non-selective action
- Sotalol: Non-selective blocker. Dose is 80–160 mg bd orally, 50–100 mg IV slowly
  - Treats ventricular tachyarrhythmias, prophylaxis of paroxysmal supraventricular tachycardias. Has class III anti-arrhythmic action
  - *Oral bioavailability,* 90%, *protein bound,* 0%; *half-life,* 10–20 hours
- Labetalol: $\alpha_1 + \beta$ blocker. Dose is 5–20 mg IV to a maximum of 200 mg. Oral dose is 400–800 mg in two divided doses
  - α_1:β::1:3 for oral, α_1:β::1:7 for IV dosing
  - *Oral bioavailability,* 25%; *protein bound,* 50%; *half-life,* 2–6 hours

Sympathomimetics

Drug	Receptor/ (μg/kg/min)	HR	Contrac-tility	SVR	DO_2	Effects
Adrena-line	$\alpha + \beta$ (0.01–0.5)	↑	↑	↑	↑	- ↑ Lactate - ↑ Renin
Noradren-aline	$\alpha_1 + \beta$ (0.05–0.5)	↓	↑	↑	↑	- Extravasation can cause tissue ischemia
Vasopres-sin	V_1 (0.01–0.1 U/min)	↓	↑	↑	↑	- In diabetes insipi-dus as well
Dopamine	$D_1 + D_2$ (1–5) β (5–10) α (>10)	↑	↑	↑/↓	↑	- Splanchnic dilation - Extrapyramidal movement - Nausea and vomiting
Dobuta-mine	$\beta_1 + \beta_2$ (0.5–20)	↑	↑	↓	↑	- No effect on splanchnic vessels
Dopex-amine	β_2, D_1 (0.5–6)	↑	↑	↓	No	- ↑ Renal and splanchnic blood flow
Isoprena-line	$\beta_1 + \beta_2$ (0.5–10 μg/ min)	↑	↑	↓	↑	- ↑ Renal and splanchnic blood flow
Ephedrine	$\alpha + \beta$	↑	↑	↑	↑	- Indirect sympatho-mimetic (noradrena-line release from nerves)
Meta-raminol	α_1 + some β	↓	↑	↑	↑	- Tachyphylaxis
Phenyl-ephrine	α_1	↓	↑	↑	↑	- Used in obstetrics as better cord arterial blood gas (ABG) profile
Enoxim-one	PDE III inhibitor (5–20)	↑	↑	↓	No	- Takes 30 min to act - $T_{1/2}$: 7.5 hours - ↑ AV conduction

(*Continued*)

Drug	Receptor/ (μg/kg/min)	HR	Contrac-tility	SVR	DO_2	Effects
Milrinone	PDE III inhibitor (0.375–0.75)	↑	↑	↓	No	- Pulmonary vasodilation - Used in right heart failure
Levosi-mendan	Ca^{2+} sensitizer (0.05–0.2)	↑	↑	↓	No	- Stabilises troponin C and actin myosin cross bridges

- Glucagon and theophylline also increase myocardial contractility
- Ephedrine causes tachyphylaxis due to depletion of neurotransmitter stores

Antiplatelet agents

- **Classification:** Treatment and prevention of arterial clots
  - **Cyclooxygenase (COX) inhibitors:** Aspirin
  - **Adenosine diphosphate (ADP) receptors/P2Y$_{12}$ receptor inhibitors:** Clopidogrel, ticlopidine, prasugrel, ticagrelor
  - **Phosphodiesterase inhibitors:** Dipyridamole
  - **GPIIb/IIIa inhibitors:** Abciximab, tirofiban, eptifibatide
- **Clopidogrel:** Prodrug that requires CYP450 for activation
  - Competitive antagonist. Irreversibly binds to P2Y$_{12}$ receptor of platelet
  - Metabolised by many genetic variants of CYP2C19, resulting in variable antiplatelet effects
  - Used for prevention of thrombotic events in peripheral vascular disease and along with aspirin for ST-segment elevation myocardial infarction (STEMI) and non-ST-elevation myocardial infarction (NSTEMI)
  - 300-mg loading dose followed by 75-mg maintenance dose
- **Prasugrel:** Prodrug but less susceptible to genetic variants of CYP450
  - Competitive antagonist. Irreversibly binds to P2Y12 receptor of platelet
  - Faster acting than clopidogrel but associated with more serious bleeding
  - Used in percutaneous coronary intervention (PCI) in acute coronary syndrome and continued for 12 months with aspirin
- **Ticagrelor:** Reversible noncompetitive allosteric antagonist of ADP receptor
  - Used in PCI in acute coronary syndrome and continued for 12 months with aspirin

- **Dipyridamole:** Inhibits cellular uptake of adenosine, potentiates the effects of prostacyclin and at high doses inhibits platelet phosphodiesterase activity
  - Coronary artery vasodilator
- **Abciximab:** Monoclonal antibody
  - Plasma half-life of 20 min but residual effect for 15 days
- **Eptifibatide:** Dose is 180 µg/kg, then by IV infusion, µg/kg/min for up to 72 hours
  - Plasma half-life of 200 min

Drug	Time before puncture/ Catheter manipulation or removal	Time after puncture/ Catheter manipulation or removal
Aspirin/non-steroidal anti-inflammatory drugs (NSAIDs)	None	None
Dipyridamole	No additional precautions	No additional precautions
Clopidogrel	7 days	6 hours
Ticlopidine	10 days	6 hours
Prasugrel	7–10 days	6 hours
Ticagrelor	5 days	6 hours
Abciximab	48 hours	6 hours
Tirofiban	6–8 hours	6 hours

Anticoagulants

- **Classification:** Treatment and prevention of venous clots
  - Oral: Includes newer oral anticoagulants
    - **Direct factor Xa inhibitor:** Apixaban, edoxaban, rivaroxaban
    - **Direct thrombin inhibitor:** Dabigatran
    - **Indirect vitamin K antagonists:** Warfarin
  - Parenteral: Can be given subcutaneously or IV
    - **Direct factor Xa inhibitor:** Otamixaban
    - **Direct thrombin inhibitor:** Argatroban, bivalirudin
    - **Indirect agents:** unfractionated heparin (UFH), low molecular weight heparin (LMWH) and fondaparinux

- **Reversal of anticoagulants**
  - ○ **Protamine sulphate:** UFH nullified by it. It is a highly positive molecule that binds to a negatively charged heparin molecule
    - ✦ Allergic reaction in those having fish allergies, diabetes and vasectomised men. Can cause pulmonary hypertension
    - ✦ Dose is 1 mg protamine to nullify 100 U of UFH. Given slowly to avoid hypotension at 5 mg/min. Maximum dose is 50 mg
  - ○ **Prothrombin complex concentrate:** Factors II, VII, IX and X with protein C and S harvested from blood
    - ✦ 25–50 units/kg. Faster reversal (10 min) and less volume required than fresh frozen plasma (FFP)
- **Apixaban:** Prophylaxis of recurrent pulmonary embolism, venous thromboembolism following knee and hip replacement surgery, stroke and systemic embolism in non-valvular atrial fibrillation
  - ○ Treatment of pulmonary embolism
- **Edoxaban:** Prophylaxis of recurrent pulmonary embolism, stroke and systemic embolism in non-valvular atrial fibrillation
  - ○ Treatment of pulmonary embolism
- **Dabigatran:** Prophylaxis of recurrent pulmonary embolism, venous thromboembolism following knee and hip replacement surgery, stroke and systemic embolism in non-valvular atrial fibrillation. Used in patients with moderate renal failure and increased risk of bleeding
  - ○ Treatment of pulmonary embolism
- **Rivaroxaban:** Prophylaxis of recurrent pulmonary embolism, venous thromboembolism following knee and hip replacement surgery, stroke and systemic embolism in non-valvular atrial fibrillation
  - ○ Prophylaxis of atherothrombotic events in patients with coronary artery disease or symptomatic peripheral artery disease at high risk of ischaemic events (in combination with aspirin)
  - ○ Treatment of pulmonary embolism
- **Argatroban:** Anticoagulation in patients with heparin-induced thrombocytopenia type II who require parenteral antithrombotic treatment
- **Fondaparinux: Indirect inhibitor of factor Xa**
  - ○ Prophylaxis of venous thromboembolism in patients after undergoing major orthopaedic surgery of the hip or leg, or abdominal surgery and medical patients immobilised because of acute illness
  - ○ Treatment of deep vein thrombosis (DVT), pulmonary embolism, angina and myocardial infarction

	Unfractionated heparin	Low molecular weight heparin	Warfarin
Mechanism of action	- 5000–25,000 Da - Binds to antithrombin III more than Xa inhibition - IX, X, XI and XII are inhibited	- 2000–8000 Da - Xa inhibition more than antithrombin III binding	- Inhibits synthesis of vitamin K-dependent clotting factors II, VII, IX and X
Pharmaco-dynamics/ Side effects	- **Hypersensitivity** - Non-immune thrombocytopenia (type I): Platelets recover spontaneously - **Heparin-induced thrombocytopenia (type II): Takes 5 days** to develop, IgG antibodies against platelet factor 4 (PF4) - **Osteoporosis** - **Hyperkalaemia** - Hypotension with fast dosing	Same side effects as UFH but - Less effects on platelets - Reduced risk of HIT - Reduced need for monitoring - Single daily dose due to a longer half-life - Dose reduced in renal failure	- Haemorrhage - **Teratogenicity** during first trimester - **Fetal haemorrhage during third trimester, hence, heparin is used** - Drug interactions with NSAIDs **(plasma binding sites)**, *inhibition of metabolism* **(amiodarone, tamoxifen)**, *induction of enzymes* **(rifampicin)**
Pharmaco-kinetics	Plasma protein binding: 50% Monitoring: APTT $T_{1/2}$: 40–90 min	Plasma protein binding: 10% Monitoring: Anti-Xa $T_{1/2}$: 2–4 times that of UFH	- Plasma protein binding: 95% - Monitoring: PT-INR - $T_{1/2}$: 35–45 hours
Uses	- Infusion to prevent DVT and pulmonary embolism - During cardiopulmonary bypass - During ECMO - During vascular surgery to prevent stent occlusion	- Prophylaxis of DVT - Treatment of DVT - Treatment of acute ST-segment elevation myocardial infarction	- Prevention and treatment of DVT and pulmonary embolism

(Continued)

	Unfractionated heparin	Low molecular weight heparin	Warfarin
Dose	Treatment of pulmonary embolism: Loading dose 75 U/kg followed by infusion of 18 U/kg/hr	- Prophylaxis of DVT - 1 mg/kg OD - Treatment of DVT - 1 mg/kg BD, 1.5 mg/kg OD	- 3–9 mg/day

Drug	Time before puncture/ Catheter manipulation or removal	Time after puncture/ Catheter manipulation or removal
Unfractionated heparin	4–6 hours	1 hour
LMWH (prophylaxis)	12 hours	4 hours
LMWH (treatment)	24 hours	4 hours
Warfarin	INR <1.5	After catheter removal
Fondaparinux	36–42 hours	6–12 hours
Rivaroxaban	22–26 hours	4–6 hours
Apixaban	26–30 hours	4–6 hours
Dabigatran	Contraindicated	6 hours
Argatroban	4 hours	2 hours

Tranexamic acid

- Synthetic derivative of lysine
- **Mechanism of action:** Competitively inhibits activation of plasminogen to plasmin. At higher concentrations becomes a non-competitive inhibition of plasminogen
- **Pharmacokinetic (PK) properties**
  - **Absorption:** 30–50% oral bioavailability
  - **Volume of distribution:** 0.18 L/kg
  - **Plasma protein binding:** 3%
  - **Route of elimination:** 95% of drug excreted unchanged in urine
  - **Half-life:** Elimination half-life is 2 hours and terminal half-life is 11 hours
- **Side effects:** Hypotension, metallic taste, fever, nausea, diarrhoea

- Clinical Uses
  - **Trauma patients (CRASH-2 trial):** 1 g STAT followed by 1 g over 8 hours
  - Traumatic brain injury (TBI) patients (CRASH-3 trial): Tranexamic acid safe in TBI. Treatment within 3 hours reduces head injury-associated deaths
  - Postpartum haemorrhage

Diuretics

- **Classification of diuretics**
  - **Proximal convoluted tubule (PCT):** Carbonic anhydrase inhibitors, e.g., acetazolamide
  - **Loop of Henle:** Loop diuretics, e.g., furosemide, **bumetanide**
  - **Distal convoluted tubule (DCT):** Thiazides, e.g., bendroflumethiazide
  - **Collecting duct (CD):** Potassium-sparing diuretics, e.g., spironolactone, amiloride, triamterene (cause hyperkalaemia)
  - Osmotic diuretics, e.g., mannitol

	Furosemide	**Bendroflumethiazide**
Mechanism of action	- Acts on Na^+-K^+-Cl^- cotransporter on thick **ascending loop of Henle** - Inhibits absorption of Na^+, K^+ and Cl^- ions	- Acts on Na^+-K^+ cotransporter on **distal convoluted tubule** - Inhibits absorption of Na^+ and Cl^- ions
Pharmaco-dynamic/ Side effects	- CVS: ↓ Preload, ↓ SVR - Biochemistry: ↓ Na^+, ↓ Cl^-, ↓ K^+, ↓ H^+, ↓ Mg^{2+}, ↑ Ca^{2+}, ↑ uric acid - Renal: ↑ GFR (used in low GFR) - Hyperglycaemia, Hypercholesterolemia - **Ototoxicity:** Rapid injection and reversible - ↑ Lithium levels	- CVS: ↓ Preload, ↓SVR - Biochemistry: ↓ Na^+, ↓ Cl^-, ↓ K^+, ↓ H^+, ↓ Mg^{2+}, ↑ Ca^{2+}, ↑ **uric acid** - Renal: ↓ GFR - **Hyperglycaemia**, Hypercholesterolemia - Blood dyscrasias: anaemia, leucopenia and thrombocytopenia - Impotence - Pancreatitis
Pharmaco-kinetics	- Bioavailability: 65% - Protein binding: >95% - Excreted unchanged in urine	- Oral bioavailability: 100% - Protein binding: 96% - $T_{1/2}$: 9 hours

(Continued)

	Furosemide	Bendroflumethiazide
Uses	- Congestive heart failure - Pulmonary oedema - Forced diuresis in AKI	- Hypertension - Congestive heart failure
Dose	- 20–160 mg depending upon refractory oedema	- 2.5–5 mg OD orally

Loop diuretics have the highest efficacy amongst all the diuretics. However, they increase urinary sodium but not as high as atrial natriuretic peptide (ANP), which causes increased urinary sodium and increased urine output.

	Spironolactone	Acetazolamide	Mannitol
Mechanism of action	- Acts on DCT and collecting duct - Competitive antagonist of aldosterone	- Non-competitive inhibitor of carbonic anhydrase - HCO_3^- absorption at PCT is decreased	- Freely filtered by glomerulus and causes osmotic diuresis - ↑ Serum osmolality
Pharmaco-dynamic/ Side effects	- CVS: ↓ Preload, ↓ SVR - Biochemistry: ↑ Na^+, ↑ Cl^-, ↑ K^+ - Irregular menses and ↓ responses to vasopressors	- CNS: ↓ Intraocular pressure, ↓ ICP - ↓ Gastric and pancreatic secretion - ↓ Excretion of uric acid - Hyperchloraemic metabolic acidosis - **Urine becomes alkaline**	- CVS: ↓ Circulating volume - CNS: ↓ ICP, can cross BBB post-head injury and cause worsening of ICP
Pharmaco-kinetics	- Bioavailability: 70% - Protein binding: >90%	- Bioavailability: 100% - Protein binding: 70–90% - $t_{1/2}$: 6 hours	- Freely filtered at glomerulus - $t_{1/2}$: 100 min
Uses	- Hypertension - Ascites - Nephrotic syndrome - Conn's syndrome	- Mountain sickness - Glaucoma	- Reduces intracranial pressure
Dose	- 50–400 mg/day	- Oral: 250 mg to 1 g/day in divided doses - IV: 250 mg to 1 g 4 hourly	- 0.5–1 mg/kg bolus over 20 min

Antibiotics

- Gram-positive aerobic cocci
  - Staphylococci (clusters)
    - **Coagulase +ve:** *Staphylococcus aureus*
    - **Coagulase −ve:** *Staphylococcus epidermidis, Staphylococcus haemolyticus, Staphylococcus hominis*
  - Streptococci (chains)
    - **α haemolysis:** *Streptococcus pneumoniae, Streptococcus viridans*
    - **β haemolysis:** *Streptococcus pyogenes, Streptococcus agalactiae*
    - **γ haemolysis:** *Enterococci faecium, Enterococci faecalis*
- Gram-positive aerobic bacilli
  - *Nocardia*
  - *Listeria*
  - *Mycobacteria*
- Gram-positive anaerobes
  - *Clostridium*
  - *Lactobacilli*
  - *Peptostreptococcus*
  - *Propionibacterium*
- Gram-negative anaerobes
  - *Bacteroides*
  - *Fusobacterium*
- Gram-negative cocci
  - *Neisseria meningitidis, Neisseria gonorrhoea*
  - *Moraxella*
- Gram-negative coccobacilli
  - *Haemophilus influenza*
  - *Bordetella pertussis*
  - *Pasteurella*
  - *Brucella*
- Gram-negative comma shaped
  - *Campylobacter*
  - *Vibrio*
  - *Helicobacter*
- Gram-negative bacilli
  - *Escherichia coli*
  - *Klebsiella*
  - *Enterobacter, Citrobacter*

- ○ *Serratia*
- ○ *Pseudomonas*
- ○ *Proteus*
- ○ *Salmonella, Shigella*
- ○ *Acinetobacter*
- ○ *Yersinia*
- Gram-negative spirochaete
  - ○ *Treponema pallidum*
  - ○ *Leptospira*
- **Antibiotic: Inhibits bacterial cell wall synthesis**

Class	Generation	Drugs	Side effects	Bacterial activity
β-Lactams Inhibit transpeptidase Penicillins (Bactericidal)	Susceptible to β-lactamase	- Benzylpenicillin - Amoxicillin - Ampicillin	- Allergy (1–10%) - True anaphylaxis is rare (0.05%) - Small risk of cross-hypersensitivity with cephalosporins and carbapenems - Convulsions in renal impairment	Gram + cocci, most anaerobes, gramnegative cocci (***Neisseria***)
	Resistant to β-lactamase	- Co-amoxiclav (β-lactamase inhibitor clavulanic acid) - Flucloxacillin		- Community-acquired pneumonia - Skin infections
	Anti-pseudomonal	**- Piperacillin/ tazocin** (β-lactamase inhibitor tazobactam) **(IV only)**		Hospital-acquired pneumonia
β-Lactams Cephalosporins (Bactericidal)	First generation	- Cephazolin		With successive generations: - Gram +ve cover is reduced - Gram −ve cover is improved
	Second generation	- Cephalexin - Cefuroxime		
	Third generation	- Ceftriaxone - Ceftazidime		
	Fourth generation	- Cefepime		

(Continued)

Class	Generation	Drugs	Side effects	Bacterial activity
β-Lactams Carbapenem (Bactericidal)		- Imipenem - # Combined with cilastatin to prevent renal metabolism - Meropenem	- Convulsions - Post-antibiotic effect (prolonged inhibition of bacterial growth)	Broad spectrum against both gram +ve, gram -ve bacteria and anaerobic bacteria
β-Lactams Monobactams (Bactericidal)		Aztreonam	- Very little cross-hypersensitivity with penicillins and cephalosporins - Anaphylaxis	Gram -ve activity specially against *Pseudomonas*

Glycopeptides (Bactericidal) Inhibit glycopeptide synthase		- Vancomycin
		- Teicoplanin
		  - # Once daily dose possible
		  - # Better bone and cerebrospinal fluid (CSF) penetration
			- Vancomycin
			- Hypersensitivity
			- Nephrotoxicity
			- Ototoxicity
			- Neutropenia
			- Thrombophlebitis via a peripheral vein
			- Red man syndrome on rapid infusion
				- MRSA
				- *Clostridium difficile* infection

- **Antibiotics:** Inhibit bacterial protein synthesis

Action	Class	Drug	Side effects	Bacterial activity
Binds to 30S subunit of bacterial ribosomes	Aminoglycosides (Bactericidal)	- Gentamicin - Amikacin - Streptomycin (against *Mycobacterium tuberculosis*)	- Nephrotoxic (reversible) - Ototoxic (irreversible) - Muscle weakness	- Gram -ve cover - Gram +ve cover includes *Staphylococcus* - No anaerobic activity - Poor cell, CSF and sputum penetration

(*Continued*)

Action	Class	Drug	Side effects	Bacterial activity
	Tetracyclines (Bacteriostatic)	- Tetracycline - Doxycycline	- Gastrointestinal (GI) upset - Superinfections - Hyperpigmentation - Photosensitivity - Dental discolouration - Nephrotoxic - Leucopenia and thrombocytopenia	- Broad spectrum against both gram +ve and –ve organisms - Intracellular bacteria like *Chlamydia* and *Rickettsia* - Anti-malarial prophylaxis
	Glycylcycline (Bacteriostatic)	Tigecycline	- Nausea and vomiting	- Methicillin-resistant *Staphylococcus aureus* (MRSA) - Vancomycin-resistant enterococci (VRE) - Drug-resistant *Escherichia coli*
Binds to 50S subunit of bacterial ribosomes	Macrolides (Bacteriostatic)	- Erythromycin - Clarithromycin - Azithromycin	- GI upset - Hepatotoxicity - Ototoxicity - Thrombophlebitis on intravenous (IV) injection	- Broad spectrum against both gram +ve and –ve organisms - *Legionella, Mycoplasma* and *Chlamydia*
	Oxazolidinone (Bacteriostatic)	Linezolid (Good lung penetration)	- Thrombocytopenia - Serotonin syndrome with antidepressants	- MRSA - VRE
	Lincosamide (Bacteriostatic)	- Clindamycin - Staphylococcal joint infections	- Pseudomembranous colitis	- Serious anaerobic cover - Gram +ve cocci - *Plasmodium falciparum*

(Continued)

Action	Class	Drug	Side effects	Bacterial activity
	Bacterio-static	Chloram-phenicol	- Bone marrow suppression - Grey baby syndrome - Optic neuritis - Ototoxicity	Broad spectrum against gram +ve bacteria, gram –ve bacteria, branching bacteria (*Actinomyces*)
Forms a complex with protein elongation factor and GTP	Bacteri-cidal	- Fusidic acid - Cerebral and joint abscesses	- Abnormal liver function - Jaundice	- MRSA - *Staphylococcus epidermidis*

- **Antibiotics:** Inhibit bacterial nucleic acid synthesis

Action	Class	Drugs	Side effects	Bacterial activity
Topoisom-erase targeting	Fluoroqui-nolones (Bacteri-cidal)	- Ciprofloxacin - Levofloxacin	- *Clostridium difficile* infection - Tendonitis - Small risk of aortic dissection	- Broad spectrum against both gram +ve and -ve organisms - *Legionella, Mycoplasma, Rickettsia* and *Chlamydia*
DNA structural disruption	Imidazoles (Bacteri-cidal)	- Metronidazole - Ornidazole	- Disulfiram-like reaction with alcohol	- Obligate anaerobes-like *Clostridia* and *Bacteroides* - Protozoa such as *Trichomonas* - *C. difficile* infection
RNA poly-merase inhibition	Rifamycins (Bacteri-cidal)	- Rifampicin - Rifabutin	- Orange urine - Hepatic CYP450 inducer	- *Mycobacterium tuberculosis* - Leprosy

(Continued)

Action	Class	Drugs	Side effects	Bacterial activity
Folic acid synthesis inhibitors	Antifolates (Bacterio-static)	- Trimethoprim - Sulphon-amides	- Stevens–Johnson syndrome - Neutropenia	- Uncomplicated urinary tract infections (UTIs) - *Pneumocystis jirovecii* - *Stenotrophomonas maltophilia*

- **Antimycobacterials:** Against *Mycobacterium tuberculosis*
  - Isoniazid, rifampicin, ethambutol, pyrazinamide and streptomycin
  - **Isoniazid:** Inhibits mycolic acid synthesis. Neurotoxicity reversed by giving pyridoxine (B6) along with it
  - **Ethambutol:** Inhibits the synthesis of arabinogalactan. Side effect is optic neuritis (irreversible)
  - **Pyrazinamide:** Unknown mechanism of action. Active against intra-cellular bacilli. Can cause gout

If true allergic reactions like anaphylaxis or breathing difficulties are present, change antibiotics.

Antifungals and antivirals

- **Antifungals:** Act against moulds (*Aspergillus*) or yeasts (*Candida*)
- **Azoles:** *Inhibit lanosterol 14 α-demethylase inhibiting cell membrane* (final step of ergosterol formation)
  - Further subdivided into triazoles (fluconazole and Itraconazole) and imidazoles (ketoconazole and miconazole)
  - **Fluconazole:** First-line treatment against *Candida* infection in the stable patient
  - **Voriconazole:** First-line treatment for invasive aspergillosis and fluco-nazole-resistant *Candida* species
  - **Side effects:** Deranged liver function tests (LFTs)/hepatotoxicity, hypersensitivity, rash/pruritus
- **Polyenes:** Bind to ergosterol and create pores within the cell membrane against systemic infections
  - **Amphotericin B:** *Aspergillus, Candida* and *Cryptococcus*
    - Poor cerebrospinal fluid (CSF) and urine penetration
    - **Side effects:** Nephrotoxicity, infusion reaction, hypokalaemia, hypomagnesemia, phlebitis, reversible normocytic anaemia

- o **AmBisome:** Lipid-base formulation of amphotericin B
  - ◆ This reduces drug toxicity and improves its tolerability
- **Echinocandins:** Inhibit B-1,3-glucan synthase, e.g., caspofungin, anidulafungin
  - o Limited penetration of the BBB
  - o Treatment for azole-resistant fungal infections
  - o Empirical therapy in suspected invasive *Candida* infections in which azoles are contraindicated (unstable patient or recent azole use)
  - o Second-line agent-invasive aspergillosis (caspofungin)
  - o **Side effects:** Deranged LFTs, infusion-related reaction/thrombophlebitis, headache, flushing, rash and pruritus
- **Allylamines:** Inhibit squalene epoxidase, e.g., terbinafine
  - o Treat fungus infections of the scalp, body, groin (jock itch), feet (athlete's foot), fingernails and toenail
  - o **Side effects:** Loss of appetite, anxiety
- **Antivirals:** Act against obligate intracellular parasite
  - o **Acyclovir:** Guanine analogue. Interferes with herpes virus DNA polymerase, inhibiting viral DNA replication
    - ◆ Used against herpes simplex virus (HSV) I and II, varicella zoster virus (VZV)
    - ◆ Acyclovir is not effective against cytomegalovirus (CMV) or Epstein–Barr virus (EBV)
    - ◆ **Side effects:** Reversible acute kidney injury, deranged LFTs, CNS toxicity (tremor/confusion/fits), neuropsychiatric effects, obstructive crystalline nephropathy
  - o **Ganciclovir:** Active against CMV but more toxic than acyclovir
    - ◆ **Side effects:** Leucopenia, thrombocytopenia, anaemia, fever, rash, abnormal LFTs
  - o **Zidovudine:** Nucleoside reverse transcriptase inhibitor (NRTI). Against HIV
    - ◆ **Side effects:** Anaemia, neutropenia, deranged liver function, pigmentation of nail beds
  - o **Oseltamivir/zanamivir:** Neuraminidase inhibitors and work by reducing the replication of influenza types A and B
    - ◆ Only proven to be effective within 48 hours of symptom onset.
  - o **Foscarnet:** Pyrophosphate analogue. Inhibits viral DNA polymerase and therefore stops viral DNA replication. Used in CMV
    - ◆ **Adverse effects:** Nephrotoxicity, electrolyte disturbances

- Anti-HIV treatment
  - ○ NRTIs: For example, zidovudine, lamivudine, tenofovir, emtricitabine, abacavir
    - ◆ **Side effects:** Anaemia, neutropenia, deranged liver function, pigmentation of nail beds, pancreatitis
  - ○ **Non-nucleoside reverse transcriptase inhibitor (NNRTIs):** For example, delavirdine, nevirapine, efavirenz
    - ◆ **Side effects:** Rash, dizziness, dyslipidaemia, Stevens–Johnson syndrome, hepatic dysfunction, neuropsychiatric effects
  - ○ **Protease inhibitors:** For example, indinavir, ritonavir, lopinavir, nelfinavir, saquinavir
    - ◆ **Side effects:** Syndrome of lipodystrophy, hyperlipidaemia, diabetes mellitus type 2 and kidney stones
  - ○ **Fusion inhibitors:** Block the HIV envelope from merging with the host CD4 cell membrane, e.g., Fuzeon (enfuvirtide)
  - ○ **CCR5 receptor antagonists:** Work by attaching themselves to proteins on the surface of CD4 cells or proteins on the surface of HIV, e.g., maraviroc, ibalizumab
  - ○ **PK enhancers:** Increase the concentration of other antiretroviral drugs so that they last longer, e.g., cobicistat, ritonavir
  - ○ **Integrase strand transfer inhibitors (INSTIs):** Block the action of integrase, a viral enzyme that inserts the viral genome into the DNA of the host cell, e.g., raltegravir, elvitegravir

Hypoglycaemic agents

Insulin: Insulin is a polypeptide of 51 amino acids formed after removal of a 34-amino-acid C-peptide from pro-insulin.

- A and B chains joined by disulphide bridges
- Insulin binds to the α subunit of the insulin receptor. Insulin receptor has two α and two β subunits
- Tyrosine kinase activity is on the β subunit

Insulin type	Onset	Peak	Duration	Remarks
Rapid-acting insulin (Aspart/*lispro*/ glulisine)	20–30 min	1–3 hours	3–5 hours	5–15 min before or after meals
Short-acting insulin (Regular/*soluble insulin*)	30 min to 1 hour	2–4 hours	5–8 hours	30 min before meal

(*Continued*)

Insulin type	Onset	Peak	Duration	Remarks
Intermediate-acting insulin (*Isophane*/NPH)	2–4 hours	4–12 hours	12–18 hours	Twice-daily regimens
Long-acting insulin (*Glargine*/detemir)	1–2 hours	Flat peak	12–24 hours	Sametime every day at any time of the day

Oral hypoglycaemic agents

- **Biguanides:** Metformin acts by enhancing uptake of glucose in muscle via the GLUT-4 transporter and inhibition of hepatic and renal gluconeogenesis
  - First line of drug in pre-diabetics and type II diabetics
  - Lactic acidosis in alcohol abusers or kidney impairment
  - ***Oral bioavailability,*** 60%; ***protein binding,*** 0%. Excreted unchanged in urine
- **Sulfonylureas:** First generation, tolbutamide; second generation, gliclazide, glipizide
  - Enhances the secretion of insulin from pancreatic islet cells by binding to ATP-dependent K$^+$ channels on islet cell membranes and causing release of proinsulin
  - Added to metformin in type II diabetics
  - Tolbutamide can cause cholestatic jaundice, deranged liver function and blood dyscrasias
  - Oral bioavailability: 80%. Extensive protein binding, mostly excreted unchanged in urine
- **Meglitinides:** Repaglinide and nateglinide
  - They block the potassium channels in beta cells in the pancreas like sulfonylureas but are short acting and taken just before meals
  - Used in patients with erratic eating habits
  - ***Oral bioavailability:*** 50%. ***Plasma protein binding:*** 98%
- **Thiazolidinediones:** Pioglitazone
  - Activates peroxisome proliferator-activated receptor γ (PPARγ), increases hepatic sensitivity to insulin and improves insulin resistance
  - **Side effects:** Fluid retention, liver derangement and limb fractures
- **Dipeptidyl peptidase-4 (DPP-4) inhibitors:** Vildagliptin and sitagliptin
  - Inhibits the enzyme DPP-4 leading to increased levels of incretins

○ Side effects: Anaphylaxis, angio-oedema and Steven-Johnson syndrome

○ Sitagliptin: *Oral bioavailability:* 87%. *Plasma protein binding:* 38%

- Glucagon-like peptide-1 (GLP-1) agonist: Exenatide
  ○ Behaves as incretin and acts as agonist on GLP-1 receptor
  ○ Given as subcutaneous injections
  ○ Not recommended if creatinine clearance <30 mL/min
- Sodium-glucose cotransporter-2 (SGLT2) inhibitors: Dapagliflozin, canagliflozin, empagliflozin
  ○ SGLT2 inhibitors work by preventing the kidneys from reabsorbing glucose back into the blood
  ○ Side effects: Can lead to diabetic ketoacidosis (DKA), genital and urinary tract infections
  ○ Not recommended for prescribing to people with kidney disease
- Alpha glucosidase inhibitors: Acarbose
  ○ Inhibits intestinal alpha glucosidase, resulting in delayed absorption of glucose
  ○ Side effects: Glatulence and diarrhoea

Diazoxide is used to treat persistent hypoglycaemia and causes hyperglycaemia.

Antiemetics and prokinetics

- Classification: Based on receptors they act on
  ○ Histamine receptors H_1 antagonists: Cyclizine, cinnarizine. Used in motion sickness
  ○ Muscarinic receptor antagonist: Hyoscine, atropine. Used in motion sickness
  ○ Dopaminergic receptor D_2 antagonist: Metoclopramide, domperidone, phenothiazines, butyrophenones
    ♦ *Phenothiazines:* Prochlorperazine, chlorpromazine, promethazine
      1. Chlorpromazine: Extrapyramidal side effects, agranulocytosis, haemolytic anaemia, leucopenia
      2. *Prochlorperazine:* Extrapyramidal side effects
    ♦ *Butyrophenones:* Droperidol, haloperidol, benperidol
      1. *Droperidol:* Dissociation, dysphoria, extrapyramidal side effects, sedation, hypotension, QT_c prolongation
  ○ Serotonin receptor 5-HT$_3$ antagonist: Ondansetron, granisetron (long acting) Used with chemotherapy
  ○ Corticosteroids: Dexamethasone and methylprednisolone
  ○ Neurokinin-1 receptor antagonists: Aprepitant

- o **Cannabinoids:** Nabilone. Used with chemotherapy
- o **Propofol:** 10- to 20-mg bolus at end of surgery
- **Prokinetics: Increase gastric motility**
  - o Metoclopramide
  - o Domperidone
  - o **Erythromycin:** Acts at motilin receptors. Dose 125 mg three times a day
  - o **Neostigmine:** Acetylcholinesterase inhibitor
  - o **Cisapride:** Acts at 5-HT$_4$ receptors

Drug	Ondansetron	Cyclizine
Mechanism of action	Serotonin receptor 5-HT$_3$ antagonist	Histamine receptors H$_1$ antagonists
Pharmacodynamics/Side effects	- CVS: Bradycardia, flushing, QT$_c$ prolongation - CNS: Headache - GI: Constipation	- CVS: **Tachycardia** - GIT: ↑ Lower oesophageal tone - CNS: **Sedation** - Pain on injection
Pharmacokinetics	- Bioavailability: 80% - t$_{1/2}$: 10 hours	- Bioavailability: 60% - t$_{1/2}$: **3 hours** - **Metabolised by N-demethylation to inactive norcyclizine**
Uses	- Antiemetic	- Antiemetic - Meniere's disease
Dose	4–8 mg 8 hourly	50 mg three times a day

Drug	Metoclopramide	Domperidone
Mechanism of action	Antagonises D$_2$, 5-HT$_3$ and agonist at muscarinic receptor	Dopaminergic receptor D$_2$ antagonist
Pharmacodynamics/Side effects	- ↑ Tone of lower oesophageal sphincter - Prokinetic - Extrapyramidal side effects - Neuroleptic malignant syndrome	- ↑ Tone of lower oesophageal sphincter - Doesn't cross blood–brain barrier, hence, no extrapyramidal side effects - Galactorrhoea and Gynaecomastia
Pharmacokinetics	- Bioavailability: 30–90% - Protein binding: 18% - t$_{1/2}$: 4 hours	- Bioavailability: 15% - Protein binding: 92% - t$_{1/2}$: 7 hours

(Continued)

Drug	Metoclopramide	Domperidone
Uses	- Antiemetic - Prokinetic	- Antiemetic - Prokinetic
Dose	10 mg 8 hourly	10–20 mg 8 hourly

Drugs acting on the gastrointestinal tract

- Drugs acting on the gastrointestinal (GI) tract
  - Reduction of gastric acid secretion
    - *H_2 antagonists:* Cimetidine, ranitidine, famotidine
    - *Proton pump inhibitors:* Pantoprazole, lansoprazole, omeprazole, esomeprazole
    - *Anticholinergic drugs:* Pirenzepine, propantheline, oxyphenonium
    - *Prostaglandin analogue:* Misoprostol
  - Neutralisation of gastric acid (antacids)
    - *Systemic:* Sodium bicarbonate, sodium citrate
    - *Non-systemic:* Aluminium hydroxide, magnesium trisilicate, calcium carbonate
- H_2 antagonists: Cimetidine was the prototype drug
  - Cimetidine inhibits hepatic cytochrome P450. Other side effects are bradycardia and hypotension on rapid infusion, gynaecomastia, impotence, hallucinations, seizures
  - Ranitidine: 5% mor potent. Less CNS effects and less effects on hepatic metabolism
- Proton pump inhibitors: Omeprazole inhibits cytochrome P450 as well
  - Omeprazole oral bioavailability is 35%, lansoprazole oral bioavailability is 85% and pantoprazole oral bioavailability is 75%
- Anticholinergic drugs: Pirenzepine has been used in gastric ulcers, but side effects like dry mouth, blurred vision, constipation and difficulty in micturition in men and exacerbation of glaucoma limit its use
- Prostaglandins: Misoprostol prostaglandin E_2 analogue that is used along with NSAIDs where alternatives to NSAIDs can't be used
- Systemic antacids: 0.3 molar sodium citrate used in general anaesthesia in obstetrics patients
- Non-systemic antacids: Acid + base produces salt and water
  - Belching due to CO_2 production
  - Calcium compounds cause constipation and magnesium compounds cause laxative effect

Anticonvulsants

- **Epilepsy:** Repetitive, paroxysmal, abnormal neuronal discharges of neurons in the brain
- **Classification:** Two main mechanisms of anticonvulsants
  - Gamma-aminobutyric acid (GABA)-mediated inhibition
    - **Facilitate GABA-mediated inhibition:** Benzodiazepines, barbiturates
    - **Inhibits GABA transaminase:** Sodium valproate, vigabatrin
  - Sodium influx in nerves
    - **Blocks the inactive fast sodium channels:** Phenytoin, carbamazepine
    - **Stabilizes presynaptic sodium channels:** Lamotrigine

Drug	Phenytoin	Carbamazepine
Mechanism of action	- Binds to inactivated fast Na^+ channels decreasing flux of Na^+ into cells - Ca^{2+} and K^+ efflux also reduced	- Binds to inactivated fast Na^+ channels decreasing flux of Na^+ into cells - Ca^{2+} and K^+ efflux also reduced
Pharmaco-dynamics/ side effects	- CVS: Class 1b antiarrhythmic—Fast injection can cause hypotension - CNS: Tremors, ataxia, nystagmus, slurred speech - Hirsutism, acne, gum hyperplasia, megaloblastic anaemia, SLE - Teratogenic: Craniofacial abnormalities, mental retardation	- CVS: AV block - CNS: Sedation, Headache, diplopia, ataxia - GIT: Hepatitis - Haematology: Agranulocytosis, aplastic anaemia
Pharmaco-kinetics	- Zero-order kinetics - CYP450 inducer - Oral bioavailability: 80% - Protein binding: 90%	- CYP450 inducer - Oral bioavailability: 100% - Protein binding: 75%
Uses	- General tonic-clonic seizures - Partial seizures - Status epilepticus - 1b Antiarrhythmic - Trigeminal neuralgia	- General tonic-clonic seizures - Infantile spasms - Acute alcohol withdrawal - Trigeminal neuralgia - Diabetic neuropathy - Mood stabiliser
Doses	Seizures: IV 15 mg/kg loading followed by 100 mg 8 hourly	- 100 mg-1.6 g in 3-4 divided doses

Drug	Valproate	Levetiracetam
Mechanism of action	- Inhibits succinic semialdehyde dehydrogenase, which results in an increase in succinic semial-dehyde which acts as an inhibitor of GABA transaminase - Direct suppression of voltage-gated sodium channel activity and indirect suppression through effects on GABA	- Selective inhibition of hypersynchronised epilepti-form burst firing without affecting normal neuronal transmission, though the exact **mechanism of action is unclear** - Wide therapeutic index unlike other drugs, hence, safer to use
Pharmaco-dynamics/ Side effects	- CNS: Drowsiness - GIT: Hepatic dysfunction, Pancreatitis - Haematological: Thrombocyto-penia - Alopecia, weight gain, terato-genic	- CNS: Dizziness, psychosis, suicidal ideation - Renal: Dose reduction in severe CKD - Stevens–Johnson syndrome
Pharmaco-kinetics	- Oral bioavailability: 90–100% - Protein binding: 90% - $t_{1/2}$: 13–19 hours	- Oral bioavailability: 100% - Protein binding: 10% - $t_{1/2}$: 6–8 hours
Uses	- Absence seizures - Myoclonic epilepsy - Status epilepticus - Trigeminal neuralgia - Migraine prophylaxis - Mood stabiliser	- GTCS - Partial seizures - Myoclonic seizures
Doses	Seizures: 600 mg to 2.5 g/day in two doses	250 mg BD to 1.5 g BD orally/IV

Drug	Diazepam	Midazolam
Mechanism of action	- Agonist at the benzodiaz-epine receptor coupled to α subunit of **GABA$_A$ receptor** - Hyperpolarisation of membrane by increasing flux of Cl⁻ ions into cells	- Agonist at the benzodiazepine receptor coupled to GABA receptor. - Hyperpolarisation of membrane by increasing flux of Cl⁻ ions into cells

(Continued)

Drug	Diazepam	Midazolam
Pharmaco-dynamics/ Side effects	- CVS: ↓ VR - RR: ↓ RR - CNS: Sedation, antero-grade amnesia, tolerance and dependence	- CVS: ↓ SVR, ↑ HR - Respiratory: ↓ TV, ↑ RR - CNS: Sedation, anterograde amnesia, **ataxia** - GIT: ↓ Hepatic and renal blood flow
Pharmaco-kinetics	- Oral bioavailability: 100% - Plasma protein binding: 99% - $t_{1/2}$: >100 hours - Metabolites are active: Oxazepam, temazepam and desmethyldiazepam	- Oral bioavailability: 40% - Plasma protein binding: 95% - $t_{1/2}$: 1–4 hours - Tautomerism: If pH >4, ring closed; if pH <4 ring is open - pH: 3, pKa 8.5 - **Porphyrinogen**
Uses	- GTCS seizures - Alcohol withdrawal - Sedation, anxiolysis	- Conscious sedation - Anterograde amnesia - Anxiolysis
Doses	- IV for sedation: 5–20 mg - Alcohol withdrawal: 20–30 mg QID	- Oral: 0.5/kg, max 20 mg - IV: 0.02–0.1 mg/kg for sedation - **Can be given rectally and intranasally**

- **Lorazepam:** No active metabolites
- **Flumazenil:** Benzodiazepine antagonist with *structure similar to benzodiazepine*
  - Poor oral bioavailability hence given only IV
  - Short half-life due to hepatic metabolism. Given continuous intravenously due to shorter action than benzodiazepines
  - No recommended maximum dose. Max 5 mg needed to reverse effect of benzodiazepines

Psychoactive drugs

- **Tricyclic antidepressants:** Amitriptyline, imipramine, doxepin
  - Blocks serotonin and norepinephrine uptake on the presynaptic membrane
  - Also acts as antagonist on α_1 adrenergic, N-methyl-D-aspartate (NMDA), histamine H_1 and H_2 receptor and muscarinic receptors

o Used for treatment of depression, chronic pain

o **Side effects:** Dry mouth, blurred vision, constipation, urinary retention, sweating, increased body temperature, drowsiness, confusion, postural hypotension, tachycardia and arrhythmias (widening of the QRS complexes and QT prolongation)

o Effect of indirectly acting sympathomimetics (e.g., ephedrine and metaraminol) is potentiated by tricyclic antidepressants (TCAs)

o Avoided with directly acting sympathomimetics to prevent hypertensive crises

o Abrupt withdrawal of TCAs can lead to risk of cholinergic symptoms

- **Selective serotonin reuptake inhibitors (SSRIs):** Sertraline, fluoxetine

  o Blocks serotonin reuptake on the presynaptic membrane

  o First line of drugs used in depression

  o **Side effects:** Drowsiness, sexual dysfunction, suicidal behaviour, serotonin syndrome, bleeding (interferes with platelet function)

  o Withdrawal of SSRIs may cause dizziness, GI upset and a variety of psychiatric symptoms; hence, they should be continued on day of surgery

- **Monoamine oxidase inhibitors (MAOIs)**

  o **MAO-A:** Breaks down serotonin and norepinephrine

  o **MAO-B:** Deaminates tyramine and phenethylamine

  o **Phenelzine, tranylcypromine:** Irreversible non-specific (both A and B) MAOI

  o **Moclobemide:** Reversible MAO-A inhibitor. Used as an antidepressant

  o **Selegiline:** Irreversible MAO-B inhibitor. Used in Parkinson's disease

  o The metabolism of indirectly acting sympathomimetics (ephedrine) is inhibited, resulting in the potentiation of their action. Use direct-acting MAOIs like phenylephrine

  o **Serotonin syndrome:** Agitation, restlessness, rapid HR, high BP, high body temperature. Antidote is cyproheptadine

  o **Pethidine,** tramadol, linezolid, TCAs and lithium can precipitate **a serotonergic crisis** in patients taking MAOIs

  o Hypertension and hypertensive crises as both MAOs breakdown tyramine (aged cheese and wine) and tyramine can elevate BP

  o Irreversible MAOIs should be stopped 2 weeks before operation

  o Omitting the dose of moclobemide on the day of surgery is acceptable

- **Lithium:** Mood stabilizer and used in mania, refractory depression and cluster headaches
  - Mechanism is unknown
  - May have a role as NMDA antagonist
  - Narrow therapeutic ratio (toxicity >1.5 mmol/l) and is excreted only by kidneys
  - **Side effects:** Interference with ADH action, cardiac dysrhythmias, GI disturbances and tremor
  - Features of lithium toxicity are lethargy, restlessness, ataxia, dysrhythmias, renal failure and coma
  - Lithium is stopped at least 24 hours before surgery
- **Antipsychotics: Indicated in schizophrenia, mania and severe agitation**
  - **First generation (typical antipsychotics):** Dopamine receptor antagonists
    - Phenothiazines like chlorpromazine, prochlorperazine and butyrophenones like haloperidol
    - They also have noradrenergic, cholinergic and histaminergic blocking action
    - Side effects include extrapyramidal symptoms, sedation, prolongation of QTc interval and anticholinergic side effects
    - **Neuroleptic malignant syndrome:** Hyperthermia, severe muscular rigidity, autonomic dysfunction, ↑white blood cells (WBCs), ↑CK levels, elevated liver enzymes, myoglobinuria and acute renal failure. Antidote is dantrolene and neuromuscular blocking agents
    - Their antiadrenergic and anticholinergic effects are unpredictable; hence, other drugs with similar effects should be used with caution or avoided
  - **Second-generation (atypical antipsychotics):** Serotonin-dopamine antagonists
    - Risperidone, olanzapine, quetiapine, aripiprazole and clozapine
    - 5-HT_{2A} subtype of serotonin receptor is most commonly blocked
    - They have decreased risk of extrapyramidal side effects compared with first-generation antipsychotics. Least with quetiapine
    - They are associated with significant weight gain, postural hypotension and the development of metabolic syndrome
    - Clozapine can cause agranulocytosis and leucopoenia; therefore it requires monitoring of WBCs and absolute neutrophil count

Anti-Parkinson drugs

- Parkinsonism: Rigidity, pill-rolling tremor, bradykinesia
- Classification
  - **Dopamine precursors.** Levodopa (L-DOPA) along with a dopa decarboxylase inhibitor (DDI) like carbidopa or benserazide
    - Levodopa is converted into dopamine peripherally. Dopamine itself can't cross the BBB, so Carbidopa and benserazide (don't cross BBB) prevent peripheral decarboxylation of levodopa
    - Side effects are orthostatic hypotension, dyskinesia and hallucinations
    - Effectiveness of this treatment wanes with time. Symptom-free time is the 'on' effect. Return of hypokinesia is the 'off' effect
    - Postoperatively it can be given down a jejunal tube
  - **Dopamine receptor agonists:** Ropinirole, pramipexole, rotigotine, apomorphine and amantadine (an antiviral agent)
    - Activate postsynaptic dopamine receptors and are first-line drugs in younger patients
    - Psychiatric side effects like hallucinations, impulse control
    - Subcutaneous apomorphine and transdermal rotigotine are used as bridging therapy in patients who are unable to take or absorb antiparkinsonian medication postoperatively
  - MAOIs: Selegiline, rasagiline
    - Side effects are headache, arthralgia, exacerbation of levodopa side effects when used as adjunct
  - **Catechol-O-methyltransferase (COMT) inhibitors:** Entacapone and tolcapone
    - Side effects are dark-coloured urine, exacerbation of levodopa side effects
  - **Antimuscarinic drugs:** Orphenadrine, trihexyphenidyl, procyclidine
    - IV procyclidine is a dose of 5–10 mg is an effective treatment for acute dystonic reactions in patients given antidopaminergic reactions like metoclopramide
- Withdrawal complications of Parkinsonian drugs
  - **Parkinsonism-hyperpyrexia syndrome (PHS):** Withdrawal of levodopa
    - Neuroleptic malignant syndrome symptoms like muscle rigidity, fever, CVS instability, altered mental status
  - **Dopamine agonist withdrawal syndrome (DAWS):** Withdrawal of dopamine agonist
    - Symptoms like anxiety, nausea, depression, pain and orthostatic hypotension

Corticosteroids

Drug	Dose (mg)	Anti-inflammatory potency	Mineralocorticoid
Hydrocortisone	20	1	1
Dexamethasone	0.75	25	Minimal
Prednisone	5	4	0.25
Prednisolone	5	4	0.25
Methylprednisolone	4	5	Minimal
Cortisone	25	0.8	0.8
Aldosterone	n/a	0.3	400
Fludrocortisone	0.1	10	300

Drug	Hydrocortisone	Dexamethasone
Mechanism of action	- Naturally occurring cortisol	- Synthetic steroid
Pharmacodynamics	- CVS: Maintains vasomotor tone of small blood vessels - Respiratory: Reduces bronchial wall swelling - CNS: Mood changes	- CVS: Minimal effect - Respiratory: Decreases inflammation in aspiration pneumonitis - CNS: May cause convulsions
Side effects	Weight gain, insomnia, feeling restless, indigestion, psychosis, hirsutism, hypertension, acne, osteoporosis, low resistance to infection	
Pharmacokinetics	- Onset: 2-4 hours - Lasts: 8 hours	- Onset: 1 hour - Lasts: 4 hours
Uses	- Anaphylaxis - Sepsis	- ARDS - PONV - Cerebral oedema - High-altitude cerebral oedema - Bacterial meningitis
Dose	- Sepsis: IV 100 mg - 6–8 hourly	- Bacterial meningitis: 10 mg IV 6 hourly for 4 days. - COVID-19: 6 mg OD for 10 days - PONV: 8–16 mg daily

Uterotonics

- **Uterotonics:** Agents used to induce contraction or greater tonicity of the uterus

	Oxytocin	Ergometrine	Carboprost ($F_{2\alpha}$)
Mechanism of action	Oxytocin receptor (GPCR -G_q/phospholipase C)	Agonism of 1. Alpha-adrenergic (α_1) 2. Dopaminergic 3. Serotonin (5-HT) receptors	Prostaglandin E_2 receptor
Pharmaco-dynamics	Uterus: Uterine contractions	- Uterus: Uterine contractions - CVS: Arterial vasoconstriction by stimulation of α_1 adrenergic receptor	Uterus: Uterine contractions
Pharmaco-kinetics	- Plasma half-life: 1–6 min - Oxytocinase produced by placenta and kidney cause degradation of oxytocin and only a small percentage is excreted in the urine unchanged	- Acts quickly - IV: 1 min - IM: 7 min - Oral: 10 min - Hepatic metabolism and excreted in bile	Metabolised in the lungs and liver metabolites are excreted in urine
Side effects	- CVS: Hypotension and tachycardia, chest pain due to myocardial ischemia - GIT: Nausea and vomiting - Uterus: Hyperstimulation - Endocrine: Water intoxication by antidiuretic effect	- CVS: Severe hypertension and bradycardia, myocardial infarction - GIT: Severe nausea and vomiting, convulsions - Contraindication: Pre-eclampsia	- CVS: Sweating and flushing - Respiratory: Bronchospasm - GIT: Nausea and vomiting - CNS: Headache, dizziness - Contraindication: Asthma

(Continued)

	Oxytocin	Ergometrine	Carboprost $(F_{2\alpha})$
Clinical uses and doses	- **Induction of labour** as 0.001 U/min until 0.02 U/min - **Caesarean section:** 5 U STAT post-delivery - **Postpartum haemorrhage:** 40 U/40 mL at 10 mL/hr - **Miscarriage:** 5 U, followed by 0.02–0.04 U/min if required	- **Active management of the third stage of labour:** Combined with synthetic oxytocin 5 U IM as a dose of 500 µg following delivery - **Postpartum haemorrhage:** 5 U IM	- **Postpartum haemorrhage:** 250 µg, repeated at 15-min intervals - Total dose up to 2 mg (8 doses)

Tocolytics

- **Tocolytics:** Drugs that relax the uterus
- Indications of tocolytics
  - Prevention of premature labour
  - Cord prolapse
  - In utero resuscitation
- **Calcium channel blockers**
  - Nifedipine
  - Blocks voltage-dependent calcium channel $\rightarrow \downarrow Ca^{2+}$
  - First choice of drug for tocolysis in UK
  - **Dose:** 20–30 mg orally as loading dose followed by 10–20 mg orally every 3–8 hours, maximum of 180 mg/day
- Atosiban
  - Specific oxytocin antagonist
  - $\downarrow Ca^{2+}$
  - Given between 24 and 33 weeks of uncomplicated premature labour
  - Second choice of drug for tocolysis in UK
  - **Dose:** Initially 6.75 mg over 1 min, then IV 18 mg/hr for 3 hours, then reduced to 6 mg/hr for up to 45 hours. Maximum duration of treatment is 48 hours
- Indomethacin
  - Cyclooxygenase inhibitor
  - $\downarrow$ Prostaglandins
  - Can cause premature closure of ductal arteriosus and oligohydramnios

- ○ Ductal constriction more common after 32 weeks of gestation and 48 hours of exposure
- ○ **Dose:** 50–100 mg orally loading dose followed by 25 mg orally every 4–6 hours, maximum of 200 mg/day. Only for 48 hours
- ○ Not recommended for use in UK
- • β_2 agonists
  - ○ **Salbutamol,** terbutaline, ritodrine (discontinued)
  - ○ **Norepinephrine has no effect on uterine tone**
  - ○ ↑ cAMP → ↓ Ca^{2+} → ↓ myosin light chain kinase → smooth muscle relaxation
  - ○ **Side effects:** Tachycardia, hypertension, arrhythmias, hyperglycaemia
  - ○ National Institute of Health and Care Excellence (NICE) guidelines recommend against offering betamimetics for tocolysis
  - ○ **Dose:** Terbutaline is given in dose of 0.25 mg subcutaneously every 20–30 min for up to four doses
- • **Magnesium sulphate**
  - ○ Natural Ca^{2+} antagonist
- • **Nitrates**
  - ○ Glyceryl trinitrate, amyl nitrate
  - ○ ↑ nitric oxide → smooth muscle relaxation
- • **Volatile anaesthetics**
  - ○ Dose-dependent relaxation of smooth muscle

Non-depolarising muscle relaxants affect only skeletal muscle (not smooth muscle).

Drugs used in asthma

- • **Asthma:** Reversible bronchospasm due to smooth muscle constriction, inflammation and mucus production
- • Levels of severity of acute asthma

Stage	Findings
Moderate	- Increasing symptoms - PEFR >50–75% - No features of acute severe asthma
Severe	Any one of - PEFR 33–50% - RR >25/min - HR >110/min - Inability to complete sentences

(Continued)

Stage	Findings	
Life threatening	- Altered conscious level - Exhaustion - Arrhythmia - Hypotension - Cyanosis - Poor respiratory effort - Silent chest	- PEFR <33% - SpO_2 <92% - PaO_2 <8 kPa - Normal $PaCO_2$
Near fatal	- Raised $PaCO_2$ requiring mechanical ventilation	

- Management of chronic asthma
  - Step 1: Start short-acting β_2 agonist
  - Step 2: Add inhaled steroid
  - Step 3: Add long-acting β_2 agonist
  - Step 4: Add leukotriene receptor antagonist or slow-release theophylline
  - Step 5: Oral steroids
- Management of acute asthma
  - O_2 to maintain SpO_2 >92%
  - **Salbutamol nebulisation 2.5–5 mg back-to-back**
  - **Ipratropium nebulisation 500 µg 6 hourly**
  - Hydrocortisone 200 mg STAT followed by 50 mg 6 hourly
  - $MgSO_4$ 2 g over 20 min
  - IV salbutamol infusion at 5–20 µg/min
  - IV aminophylline bolus 5 mg/kg followed by 0.5 mg/kg/hr
  - **Adrenaline:** Nebulised or intravenous (100-µg bolus)
  - Ketamine infusion at 0.5–2 mg/kg/hr
  - Volatile anaesthetic agents

	Salbutamol	Ipratropium	Aminophylline
Mechanism of action	- β_2 agonist via cAMP - Short acting	- Muscarinic M3 antagonist - Short acting	- Competitive **phosphodiesterase inhibitor**
Effects	- CVS: Tachycardia at high doses - β_2 agonist-mediated vasodilation	- CVS: Tachycardia - GIT: Dry mouth, constipation	- CVS: Tachycardia, - Arrhythmogenic

(Continued)

	Salbutamol	Ipratropium	Aminophylline
Effects	- Metabolic: Hypoka-laemia - Uterus: Relaxes the gravid uterus	- Eye: Acute angle-closure glaucoma particularly when given with nebulised salbutamol	- CNS: ↓ Seizure threshold
Dose	- 2.5–5 mg back-to-back nebulisation - 5–20 µg/min IV	- 500 µg 6 hourly	- 5 mg/kg bolus followed by 0.5 mg/kg/hr

- **Salmeterol:** Longer acting but slow onset

Magnesium sulphate

- Fourth most abundant cation in the body. Second most intracellular cation
- **Mechanism of action**
  1. Physiological NMDA receptor antagonist
  2. Natural Ca^{2+} antagonist
  3. Inhibits presynaptic release of acetylcholine
  4. Inhibits catecholamine release
- **Pharmacodynamic actions**
  - **CVS:** Vasodilation via endothelial nitric oxide plus inhibition of catecholamine release. Decreases cardiac conduction and myocardial contractile force
  - **Respiratory:** Bronchodilation
  - **CNS:** Depresses the brain and causes sedation. Deep tendon reflexes are lost
  - **Uterus:** Relaxes uterus, used as a tocolytic
- **Magnesium toxicity**
  - **0.7–1.0 mmol/L:** Normal blood levels
  - **2–3.5 mmol/L:** Nausea and vomiting, electrocardiogram (ECG) changes
  - **4–5 mmol/L:** *Loss of tendon reflexes (Best way of monitoring toxicity)*
  - **5–7.5 mmol/L:** Respiratory paralysis
  - **10–12.5 mol/L:** Cardiac arrest

- Clinical uses
  - **Asthma:** *Used in refractory asthma:* 25 mg/kg or 2 g IV over 20 min
  - **Pre-eclampsia and eclampsia:** A loading dose of 4 g over 15 min followed by an infusion at a rate of 1 g/hr for 24 hours
  - **Fetal neuroprotection:** Magnesium sulphate to be offered to women carrying viable foetuses, who are very likely to deliver a premature baby within the next 24 hours. A loading dose of 4 g over 15 min followed by an infusion at a rate of 1 g/hr for 24 hours
  - Hypomagnesemia
  - Analgesia
  - **Arrhythmias:** Tachyarrhythmias induced by adrenaline, digitalis and bupivacaine
  - Status epilepticus

Chemotherapeutic agents

- **Classification:** Ultimate goal of chemotherapeutic agents is disruption of DNA and inhibition of proliferation of tumour cells
  - **Antimetabolites:** Act as false substrates and act as competitive inhibitors
    - Methotrexate, fluorouracil, mercaptopurine
  - **Alkylating agents:** Bind to DNA and suppress its normal function
    - Cisplatin, busulfan, chlorambucil, cyclophosphamide
  - **Antibiotics:** Topoisomerase I and II inhibitors
    - Daunorubicin, doxorubicin, camptothecins
  - **Mitotic inhibitors:** Mitotic spindle poisons
    - Vincristine and vinblastine
- **Adverse effects**
  - CVS
    - *Doxorubicin/daunorubicin:* Irreversible cardiomyopathy
    - *Cyclophosphamide/busulfan:* Endocardial fibrosis
  - **Renal:** Nephrotoxicity
    - Cisplatin
    - Methotrexate
    - Cyclophosphamide
  - **Hepatic:** Abnormal liver function
    - Cisplatin
    - Methotrexate

- Neurological
  - *Vincristine and vinblastine:* Neurotoxicity
  - *Cyclophosphamide:* Syndrome of inappropriate antidiuretic hormone (SIADH)
- Pulmonary
  - *Bleomycin:* Interstitial pneumonitis and pulmonary fibrosis
  - Methotrexate: Pulmonary fibrosis
- Haematological: Myelosuppression
  - *Methotrexate:* Anaemia
  - *Cisplatin:* Anaemia
  - Neutropenia
- **Tumour lysis 5-fluorouracil:** Hyperkalaemia, hyperphosphataemia, hypocalcaemia, hyperuricaemia

Drug toxicities

- Local anaesthetic: Onset of neurological symptoms like circumoral tingling, seizures around 6 µg/mL with CVS compromise at levels greater than 10 µg/mL
  - 20% lipid emulsion: 1.5 mg/kg bolus followed by infusion at 0.25 mL/kg/min. Two more boluses at 5-min intervals (total 3 boluses). Increase infusion rate to 0.5 mL/kg/min
- Opioid: CNS narcosis, seizures due to cerebral hypoxia
  - Naloxone titrated to effect. May have to start infusion in longer-acting opioids
- Digoxin: Nausea, vomiting, yellow vision, arrhythmias
  - Correct hypokalaemia and hypomagnesaemia
  - Phenytoin, lignocaine or amiodarone for ventricular arrhythmias
  - Digoxin-specific antibodies (Digibind)
- Paracetamol: Signs of acute liver failure like cerebral oedema, respiratory failure, renal failure, coagulation failure
  - N-acetylcysteine (NAC) effective antidote if given in 8 hours
  - Liver transplant
- Benzodiazepine: CNS narcosis
  - Flumazenil used as antagonist, can cause seizures

- **TCAs:** Myocardial depression, arrhythmias due to increased QT interval, seizures, drowsiness
  - Activated charcoal in first 24 hours
  - Bicarbonate alkalizes blood and prevents renal reabsorption
  - Lignocaine, phenytoin and magnesium for arrhythmias
- **Aspirin:** First hyperventilation due to CNS stimulatory effect and causes respiratory alkalosis and tinnitus. Then metabolic acidosis due to direct effect and causes non-cardiogenic pulmonary oedema and low Glasgow Coma Score (GCS)
  - Activated charcoal in first 24 hours
  - Bicarbonate alkalizes blood and prevents renal reabsorption
  - Haemodialysis
- **Ethylene glycol:** Hyperthermia, hypoglycaemia, hypocalcaemia, High osmolar gap metabolic acidosis
  - Ethanol to compete for metabolic pathway
  - Haemodialysis
- **Methanol:** Nausea, vomiting, GI bleeding, visual disturbances, high anion gap metabolic acidosis
  - Ethanol to compete for metabolic pathway
  - Haemodialysis

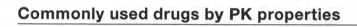

Commonly used drugs by PK properties

Drug	V_d (L/kg)
Propofol	4
Thiopentone	2.5
Ketamine	3
Etomidate	3
Alfentanil	0.6
Remifentanil	0.3
Fentanyl	4
Morphine	3.5
Pethidine	4
Codeine	5.4
Diamorphine	5
Atracurium	0.15
Cis-atracurium	0.15
Rocuronium	0.2
Lidocaine	0.7–1.5
Paracetamol	1
Warfarin	0.1–0.16
Midazolam	1.5
Penicillin	0.32–0.81

Drug	Protein bound (%)
Propofol	98
Thiopentone	80
Ketamine	25
Etomidate	75
Alfentanil	90
Remifentanil	70
Fentanyl	83
Morphine	35
Pethidine	60
Codeine	7
Diamorphine	40
Atracurium	15
Cis-Atracurium	15
Rocuronium	10
Lidocaine	70
Bupivacaine	95
Ropivacaine	94
Paracetamol	10
Aspirin	85
Diclofenac	99
Ketorolac	95
Diazepam	95
Phenytoin	95
Warfarin	99
Atenolol	5
Diltiazem	75
Gabapentin	3

Drug	Oral bioavailabilities (%)
Morphine	15–50
Fentanyl	33
Paracetamol	90
Aspirin	70
Diclofenac	50
Ibuprofen	80
Atenolol	50
Glycopyrrolate	5
Ondansetron	60
Ranitidine	50
Metoclopramide	30–90

PHYSICS

Applied Physics

13

SI Units

- Seven basic Système International (SI) units

Unit	Measure	Symbol
Second	Time	s
Metre	Distance	m
Mole	Amount	mol
Ampere	Current	A
Candela	Luminous Intensity	cd
Kilogram	Mass	kg
Kelvin	Temperature	K

- Derived SI units: Derived from SI units

Measure	Definition	Units
Speed	Metre per second	m/s
Velocity	Metre per second in a given direction	m/s
Acceleration	Metre per second squared	m/s^2
Area	Square metre	m^2
Volume	Cubic metre	m^3
Concentration	Mole per cubic metre	mol/m^3
Wave number	Reciprocal metre	m^{-1}
Current density	Ampere per square metre	A/m^2

- Derived SI units with special symbols

Measure	Name	Symbol	Units
Force	newton	N	$Kg.m/s^2$
Pressure	pascal	Pa	N/m^2
Energy/work	joule	J	N/m

(Continued)

DOI: 10.1201/9781003390244-16

Measure	Name	Symbol	Units
Power	*watt*	W	J/s
Frequency	hertz	Hz	1/s
Electrical charge	coulomb	C	A/s
Potential difference	volt	V	W/A
Capacitance	farad	F	C/V
Resistance	ohm	Ω	V/A

- Prefixes

Prefix	10^n
tera	10^{12}
giga	10^9
mega	10^6
kilo	10^3
hector	10^2
deca	10^1
	10^0
deci	10^{-1}
centi	10^{-2}
milli	10^{-3}
micro	10^{-6}
nano	10^{-9}
pico	10^{-12}
femto	10^{-15}

Definitions

- **Second:** The duration of a given number of oscillations of the caesium-133 atom
- **Metre:** The length of the path travelled by light in a vacuum during a certain fraction of a second
- **Mole:** The amount of substance which contains as many elementary particles as there are atoms in 0.012 kg of carbon-12
- **Ampere:** The current in two parallel conductors of infinite length and placed 1 m apart in a vacuum, which would produce between them a force of 2×10^{-7} N/m

- **Candela:** Luminous intensity, in a given direction, of a source that emits monochromatic light at a specific frequency
- **Kilogram:** The mass of the international prototype of the kilogram held in Sèvres, France
- **Kelvin:** 1/273.16 of the thermodynamic temperature of the triple point of water
- **Force:** What changes or tends to change the state of rest or motion of an object

  Force is measured in newtons (N), a newton being the force that will give a mass of 1 kg an acceleration of 1 metre per second per second
- **Pressure:** Pressure is the force applied over a surface

  Pressure is measured in pascal (P), a pascal is a pressure of 1 newton acting over an area of 1 square metre
- **Work:** Work is done or energy is expended whenever the point of application of a force moves in the direction of the force

  One joule of work is done when a force of 1 newton moves its point of application 1 m in the direction of the force
- **Power:** Power is the rate of working and is measured in watts

  1 watt is 1 joule per second
- **Resistance:** The unit of electrical resistance is the ohm

  The ohm is that resistance which will allow one ampere of current to flow under the influence of a potential of 1 volt
- **Capacitance:** The ability of a capacitor to store electrical charge

  A capacitor with a capacitance of 1 farad will store 1 coulomb of charge when 1 volt is applied to it

Gas laws

- **Boyle's law:** The volume of a gas varies inversely with pressure at a constant temperature

$$V \propto 1/P$$

  - *Assumes molecular size is unimportant*
- **Charles' law:** The volume of a gas varies directly with temperature at a constant pressure

$$V \propto T$$

- **Gay–Lussac's law:** The pressure of a gas varies directly with temperature at a constant volume

$$P \propto T$$

- **Avogadro's hypothesis:** Equal volumes of ideal gases at the same temperature and pressure contain equal numbers of molecules
- **Universal gas equation:** Ideal gas laws can be combined with Avogadro's hypothesis to give the equation that $PV = nRT$
- **Dalton's law of partial pressure:** *Pressure exerted by a single gas in a mixture of gases is the same as that which it would exert if it alone occupied the container*

Other laws

- **Fick's law:** The rate of diffusion of a substance across a surface is directly proportional to the concentration gradient
- **Graham's law:** The rate of diffusion of a gas is inversely proportional to the square root of its molecular weight
- **Raoult's law:** The reduction of vapour pressure of a solvent is proportional to the molecular concentration of the solute
- **Henry's law:** The amount of a gas dissolved in a given liquid is directly proportional to the partial pressure of the gas in equilibrium with the liquid at a particular temperature

\# Rate of diffusion is inversely proportional to membrane thickness.

\# Ambient pressure does not affect rate of diffusion.

Flow

- **Flow:** Flow is the amount of a liquid or a gas passing a given point per unit time
- **Laminar flow:** Fluid moves so that the molecule in the substance always maintains a constant spatial relationship to all the others that are flowing in the same direction
  - No eddies or turbulence
  - Flow at centre is twice as much compared with the flow at side of tube
  - **Hagen–Poiseuille equation:** $\text{Flow} = \dfrac{\prod \times \Delta P \times r^4}{8 \times L \times \eta}$

    where $\prod = \text{Pi} = 3.14$

    $\Delta P = $ Change in pressure

    $r = $ Radius

    $L = $ Length of tube

    $\eta = $ Viscosity

- **Turbulent flow:** Fluid flows in a way the orderly management of the molecules is lost
  - Eddies and swirls
  - Angles and constrictions can cause laminar flow to convert into turbulent flow
  - **Turbulent flow is proportional to $\sqrt{P}$, r^2, $1/\sqrt{L}$, $1/\sqrt{\rho}$**

    where P = Pressure

    r = Radius

    L = Length of tube

    ρ = Density

- **Reynold's number:** Number that predicts if a fluid will have a turbulent or laminar flow
  - Reynolds number <2000 predicts laminar flow whereas Reynolds number >2000 predicts turbulent flow
  - **Reynold's number $= \dfrac{v \times \rho \times D}{\eta}$**

    where v = Velocity of fluid

    ρ = Density

    D = Diameter of tube

    η = Viscosity

- **Bernoulli principle:** An increase in the speed of a fluid occurs simultaneously along with a decrease in pressure

- **Venturi effect:** Drop in pressure due to increase in speed of a fluid through a narrow orifice to entrain a second gas. Used in venturi face masks, nebulisers, suction devices, testing Bain circuit, scavenging systems, etc.

- **Coanda effect:** Fluid particles often adhere to flat and curved surfaces due to a pressure difference that exists between the top and bottom sides of the particles; this tendency to adhere is known as the Coanda effect. For example, it is so hard to pour liquid from a mug without spilling

- **Critical velocity:** Velocity above which the flow of a fluid within a tube change from laminar to turbulent flow

- **Heliox:** This is 21% oxygen and 79% helium. Helium is lighter than nitrogen when comparing density. Therefore, *reduction in density* changes the flow of mixture from turbulent to laminar flow, decreasing the work of breathing

- For fast volume resuscitation, a 14–G cannula in the anterior cubital fossa (1:30 min) or a pulmonary artery catheter (PAC) sheath (1:05 min) in the femoral vein are fast enough, but it is easier to put in a cannula for resuscitation

- **Fluid flow is maximally affected by radius as flow $\sim R^4$**

Osmosis

- **Osmosis:** Movement of water molecules (solvent) across a semi-permeable membrane, from a dilute solution to a concentrated solution
- **Diffusion:** Movement of solute molecules from a high concentration to a low concentration
- **Osmolarity:** Number of osmoles of solute per litre of solution. Affected by temperature
- **Osmolality:** Number of osmoles of solute per kilogram of solution. Not affected by temperature. Osmolality = [2 × Na$^+$] + [Glucose] + [Urea] = 290 mOsm/kg
- **Tonicity:** Relative osmolality between two fluid compartments
- **Osmotic pressure:** Pressure required to stop the net movement of water by osmosis across a semi-permeable membrane
- Colloid osmotic pressure (oncotic pressure): *Electrolytes contribute to more than 99% of osmolality and osmotic pressure.* Plasma proteins like albumin contribute to remaining 1%, which is known as oncotic pressure ~25–30 mm Hg. Oncotic pressure is the major determinant of movement of fluid across capillaries. Albumin is responsible for 75% of oncotic pressure
- **Measurement of osmotic pressure (osmometer):** Osmometers use Raoult's law that *1 mol of a solute when added to 1 kg of water will depress the freezing point by 1.86°C.* Colligative properties are

  1. Vapour pressure lowering
  2. Boiling point elevation
  3. Melting point depression
  4. Osmotic pressure

- **Osmoregulation:** Body has osmoreceptors in the anterior hypothalamus. These receptors are outside the blood–brain barrier. They respond to osmolality changes and secrete antidiuretic hormone (ADH; vasopressin)
  - ADH acts on V2 receptors on collecting ducts leading to increased water absorption
  - ADH acts on V2 and releases factor VIII from the endothelium
  - ADH acts on V1 causing platelet aggregation and degranulation
  - ADH stimulates thirst
  - ADH causes arteriolar vasoconstriction
  - **ADH causes glycogenolysis**

- Water regulation: Three main factors are involved
  o Osmoreceptors sense increased osmolality, release ADH which stimulates thirst
  o Renin-angiotensin-aldosterone senses volume depletion and causes aldosterone secretion which retains Na^+ and water
  o Dry pharynx stimulates thirst

Diathermy

- Diathermy (Bovie machine): Device used to cut or coagulate tissue
- Principle: Based on *current density.* If a current is applied over a small area, the density would be high and heating will occur. Conversely, when the same amount of current is applied over a large area, the density will be less and no heating occurs
- 0.5–1 MHz is the diathermy frequency: Electricity has potential to cause ventricular fibrillation (VF) depending on its frequency. The peak potential to cause VF occurs at ~ 50 hz (Mains frequency)
- Problems with diathermy
  o *Burns* if monothermic diathermy plate not properly adherent to skin
  o Interference with monitors
  o Interference with pacemaker
- Types of diathermies
  o *Monopolar:* One small and one big electrode. Small, pointed electrode has high current density for cutting and coagulation. Big electrode is large plate connected to a fixed point like a leg. *The modern diathermy return plate is not connected directly to earth*
  o *Bipolar:* This typically uses a pair of forceps with an electrode on each of the prongs
    * Less powerful
    * Preferred in patients with pacemaker
- Patterns of diathermy
  o *Cutting:* High energy delivered continuously at high frequency. Alternating sine wave pattern
  o *Coagulation:* Energy given in bursts. Damped wave pattern. Coagulation modes are only active <10% of the time
- A capacitor is put in the lead from the diathermy to earth. The capacitor gives a high impedance to main frequency current and prevents patient injury by preventing current flow

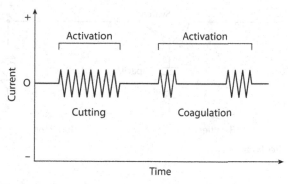

Figure 13.1   Diathermy wave.

Defibrillators

- **Resistance:** Opposition to flow of direct current (DC) (ohms [Ω])
- **Reactance:** Opposition to flow of alternating current (AC) (Ω)
- **Impedance:** Total of resistance plus reactance of opposition to electrical flow (Ω)
  - Skin: 2000 Ω. Decreases with wet hands
  - Thoracic impedance: 50–150 Ω
  - Body tissue: 500 Ω
  - Shoes: 200,000 Ω
- **Capacitance:** Ability of a capacitor to store electrical charge (farads [F])
  - *Potential difference across a capacitor decreases as AC frequency increases because impedance is inversely proportional to AC frequency*
- **Inductance:** Ability to generate a resistive force under the influence of changing current (henry [H])
- **Defibrillator:** Delivers DC shock to heart as AC causes myocardial damage
  - A rectifier is used to derive DC power from AC power
  - A step-up transformer increases the mains voltage from 240 V to 5000 V
  - A capacitor is used to store charges. They have low reactance to AC but high resistance to DC
  - An inductor is used to prolong the duration of current discharge. A magnetic flux is induced whenever a current flows through the coils causing a back electromagnetic field (EMF) and prolongs the charge. Inductor has high reactance to AC but low resistance to DC

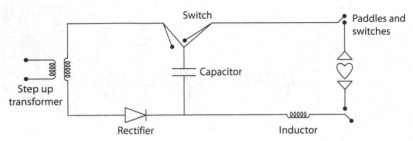

Figure 13.2 Defibrillator.

- o During charging, current just flows through the capacitor plates, which store the charge
- o **When discharging, the stored charge from the capacitor is now delivered to the patient. The inductor prolongs the effective delivery of current to myocardium**
- • Types of defibrillators
  - o **Monophasic:** Current flows in one direction only from one electrode to another
  - o **Biphasic: Current flows in alternating directions. It lowers the energy levels required, reducing risk of burns and myocardial damage**

Electricity

- • **Current:** Current is a flow of electrical charge carriers, usually electrons or electron-deficient atoms
  - o DC: Constant in direction of flow
    - • Magnitude can be measured directly
  - o **AC: Direction of flow changes repeatedly and regularly reverses direction**
    - • Sinusoidal pattern
    - • Easier and cheaper to generate
    - • Easier to transform like changing voltage and current
    - • Easier to convert AC to DC. Placing a one-way valve in a current direction known as a DIODE
    - • Measurement of the average voltage of a sinusoidally varying AC will yield zero as forward and reverse currents cancel each other out
    - • **Root mean square (RMS) voltage:** 240 V RMS. So to measure AC voltage we square, calculate mean and then get a square root result (root of the mean of the squared value)

- **Effective voltage:** ±339 V. The equivalent DC voltage or current which would dissipate the same amount of power in a resistor
- AC at household frequency of 50 Hz is more dangerous than bigger frequencies like 100 kHz

- **Power production**
  - ○ **Single-phase alternator:** When a wire is exposed to a fluctuating magnetic field a voltage is induced that tries to move charge already present in the wire producing current if a circuit existed
    - If the wire and magnet are rotated relative to each other than the voltage induced in the wire will vary sinusoidally with time producing AC
  - ○ **Three-phase alternators:** It is more efficient to spin a magnetic field within three coils of wire
    - A sinusoidally varying voltage is induced in all three coils, but the current produced is asynchronous
  - ○ **Transformer:** Current in a wire produces a magnetic field and adjacent fields interact to generate a force
    - A transformer consists of two coils linked only by a magnetic field
    - The passage of an AC through one coil will produce a sinusoidally varying magnetic field
    - The second coil is exposed to this varying field and as a consequence a voltage and current are induced in this coil
    - The induced voltage in this second coil depends upon the voltage applied to the first coil and the ratio of the number of turns forming the first and second coils

- **Power transmission:** In a power station a magnetic field is rotated past a set of three coils in a three-phase alternator
  - ○ **Power station:** Three output wires carrying the three phases leave the power station at very high voltage (275 kV)
  - ○ **Local transformer:** Power arrives at a local transformer at 11 kV after voltage is reduced by a series of step-down transformers
  - ○ **Electricity substation:** Voltage is reduced to 250 V, so one of the wires with 250 V supplies the household while the other point of the same wire will be earthed
    - *Star point:* When one end of all the three wires is connected to earth
    - Therefore, the wire coming to house is called LINE (brown in colour). The wire connected to earth as the electricity substation is called NEUTRAL (blue in colour)
    - The neutral line connected to EARTH at ELECTRICITY SUBSTATION protects the HOUSE should lightning strike the overhead power lines

- But if a piece of equipment at home develops a fault and current escapes to the metallic case, if you touch the apparatus while touching the earth, you will complete the circuit due to the star point also earthing at the substation
- *Local earth connection:* So, another earthing point apart from star point earthing is established close to your house known as a local earth connection (green/yellow in colour)
- Now if a current will come to the metallic case of a faulty equipment, current will pass through both you and the local earth connection but the proportion which passes through you depends on your resistance compared with that of the local earth connection
  - o Requirements of earth connection: Local earth connection must have a low enough resistance so that almost all the current escapes you
    - Leakage current <0.5 mA
    - Impedance < 0.1 Ω
    - Earth surge test: 25 A for 5 s
  - o A single earthing point is used for all electrical equipment connected to the patient as it prevents current flow through the patient.

Electrical safety

- Mechanism of patient injury
  - o Electric shock
    - Macroshock
    - Microshock
  - o Burns
    - Direct heating
    - Fire
    - Explosions
  - o Interference
    - Monitoring
    - Therapeutic equipment
- Macroshock: Occurs when current passes through the body via contact with the skin
  - o 1 mA → tingling
  - o 5 mA → Pain
  - o 15 mA → Severe pain and muscle spasm (no let go)
  - o 50 mA → Respiratory muscle spasm
  - o 100 mA → VF

- **Microshock:** Occurs when invasive patient connections are placed across or in close proximity to myocardial tissue
  - 50–100 μA of current directly to the ventricle can induce VF
- **Types of electrical equipment based on grade of protection they offer**
  - *Class I:* The casing of equipment is **connected to earth.** So basic protection only
  - *Class II:* Double layer of casing to double insulate electrical parts from the user
    - With the advent of plastic equipment, this is now the most common type
    - No earthing required
  - *Class III:* **They receive power through an isolating transformer or a battery**
    - These are devices with a 'floating circuit'
    - This means the circuit has no direct connection with the mains supply
    - Safety extra low voltage (SELV) which <24 V AC
    - Can still cause microshocks but still preferred as it avoids AC current
- **Types of electrical equipment based on current they leak**
  - *Type B:* Approved for body (B) connections. Low leakage currents
    - 0.5 mA for class I and 0.1 mA for class II
  - *Type BF:* Same as type B except that the piece of equipment that is applied to the patient is isolated from all the other parts
  - *Type CF:* Approved for cardiac (C) connections. Lowest leakage currents
    - 0.05 mA for class I and 0.01 mA for class II

  Types B, BF and CF can all be provided with defibrillator protection.
- **Electrical safety devices**
  - Fuses: Simple pieces of wire in series with the live connection of a circuit
    - When current flows through the piece of wire it heats up
    - If a certain current is exceeded then the fuse will melt, shutting off the supply current
  - Earth leakage circuit breakers (ELCBs): Can be used instead of fuse
    - Unlike a fuse, which operates once and then must be replaced, a circuit breaker can be reset
    - Works on the principle of electromagnetism
    - The electricity magnetizes the electromagnet and boosts the electromagnet's magnetic force
    - When the current jumps to unsafe levels, the electromagnet is strong enough to pull down a metal lever connected to the switch linkage and shuts off electricity

- o Isolating transformer (floating circuit): Equipment supplying the patient is supplied via an extra transformer connected to mains
  - ◆ This transformer has no earthing; hence, the dangers of mains because of earthing are circumvented by putting another transformer between the patient and mains
- o Line isolation monitor (LIM): Now even an isolating transformer can develop a fault and accidently get connected to earth. So, we put another piece of equipment between the isolating transformer and the patient. This is called the line isolation monitor
  - ◆ It generates an alarm if an earth connection is made
  - ◆ Doesn't switch off supply if an electric surge happens, just alarms are activated
- Interference with monitoring and therapeutic equipment
  - o Electromagnetic induction
    - ◆ Current needs to be switched on
    - ◆ As current flows through the wire, electromagnetic field will transfer energy to nearby conductors, acting like an inefficient TRANSFORMER
    - ◆ Magnetic field strength varies as the reciprocal of the separation squared
    - ◆ Battery powered equipment is equally affected
    - ◆ Screened cable doesn't prevent magnetic field
  - o Electrostatic induction
    - ◆ Current doesn't need to be switched on
    - ◆ Potential difference is there but no current is flowing
    - ◆ Wires can act as a CAPACITOR plate
    - ◆ Can be prevented by a screened cable

The ultimate goal of electrical safety is to avoid earth leakage currents.

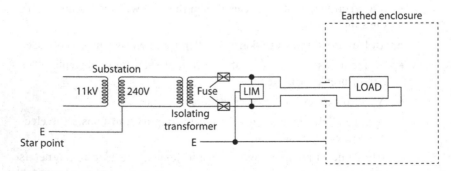

Figure 13.3 Isolating transformer.

Electrical symbols

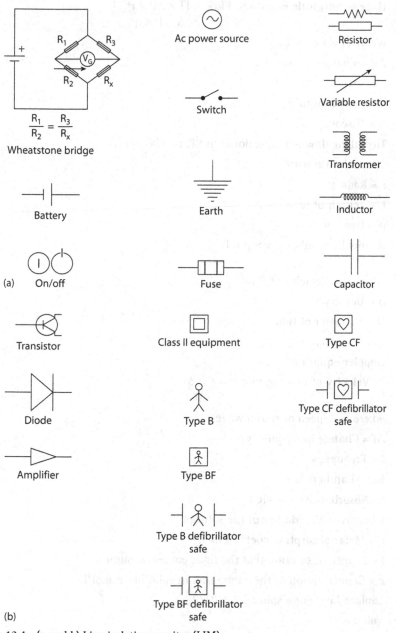

$$\frac{R_1}{R_2} = \frac{R_3}{R_x}$$

Wheatstone bridge

Ac power source

Resistor

Switch

Variable resistor

Battery

Earth

Transformer

Inductor

(a) On/off

Fuse

Capacitor

Transistor

Class II equipment

Type CF

Diode

Type B

Type CF defibrillator safe

Amplifier

Type BF

Type B defibrillator safe

Type BF defibrillator safe

(b)

Figure 13.4   (a and b) Line isolation monitor (LIM).

Formulas used in physics

- **Hagen–Poiseuille equation:** $\text{Flow} = \dfrac{\Pi \times \Delta P \times r^4}{8 \times L \times \eta}$

  where Π = Pi = 3.14

  ΔP = Change in pressure

  r = Radius

  L = Length of tube

  η = Viscosity

- **Turbulent flow** is proportional to $\sqrt{P}$, r^2, $1/\sqrt{L}$, $1/\sqrt{\rho}$

  where P = Pressure

  r = Radius

  L = Length of tube

  ρ = Density

- **Reynold's number** = $\dfrac{v \times \rho \times D}{\eta}$

  where v = Velocity of fluid

  ρ = Density

  D = Diameter of tube

  η = Viscosity

- **Doppler equation**
  - Velocity of moving target = $\dfrac{c \times \Delta f}{2f}$

  where c = Speed of sound wave

  Δf = Change in frequency

  f = Frequency

- **Beer–Lambert law**
  - Absorbance (A) = $\varepsilon l c$

  where A = Absorbance of the solution

  ε = Molar absorption coefficient

  l = Length of solution that the light passes through

  c = Concentration of the compound in solution in mol/L

- **Laplace law:** For a sphere, P = 2T/R

- **Voltage**

$$V = IR$$

where V = Voltage, I = Current, R = Resistance

$$Q = CV$$

where Q = Charge, C = Capacitance, V = Voltage

$$E = 1/2QV$$

where E = Energy, Q = Charge, V = Voltage

$$P = IV$$

where P = Power, I = Current, V = Voltage

- **Resistance:** In series,

Total resistance $= R_1 + R_2$

  ○ In parallel,

Total resistance $\dfrac{1}{R} = \dfrac{1}{R_1} + \dfrac{1}{R_2}$

- **Bernoulli principle:** An increase in the speed of a fluid occurs simultaneously along with a decrease in pressure

- **Venturi effect:** Drop in pressure due to increase in speed of a fluid through a narrow orifice to entrain a second gas. Used in venturi face masks, nebulisers, suction devices, testing Bain circuit, scavenging systems, etc.

- **Coanda effect:** Fluid particles often adhere to flat and curved surfaces due to a pressure difference that exists between the top and bottom sides of the particles; this tendency to adhere is known as the Coanda effect. For example, It is so hard to pour liquid from a mug without spilling

Clinical Measurement

14

Biological potentials

- **Biological potentials:** Records of a biological event such as a beating heart, ticking brain or a contracting muscle
  - Depending upon cell type, signals differ in terms of their frequency and voltage
- **Heart signals:** *Electrocardiogram (ECG),* voltage 1–2 mV; frequency 0.05–100 Hz
- **Skeletal muscle signals:** *Electromyograph (EMG),* voltage 100–30 mV; frequency 1–20,000 Hz
- **Brain:** *Electroencephalogram (EEG),* voltage 10–300 μV, frequency depends upon wave
  - α wave: 8–13 Hz
  - β wave: >13 Hz
  - δ wave: 0–4 Hz
  - θ wave: 4–8 Hz
- **Components of a machine showing bio signals:** A detection device (electrodes), a transducer, an amplifier and a display device (monitor)
- **Transducer:** A transducer **converts a signal in one form of energy to a signal in another**
  - Transducer can be active (piezoelectric) or passive (strain gauge)
  - Can be used to measure temperature
- **Amplifiers:** An amplifier is a device which increases the amplitude of an electrical current/signal using a power supply
  - **A differential amplifier:** Electronic amplifier that amplifies the difference between two input voltages but suppresses any voltage common to the two inputs known as common mode rejection
- **Filters:** Despite common mode rejection, some interference may still be present in the signal to be amplified
  - *High-pass filters:* Eliminates all Currents with low frequency
  - *Low-pass filters:* Eliminates all Currents with high frequency
  - *Notch filter:* Rejects a specific band of frequencies

DOI: 10.1201/9781003390244-17

- Interference
  - Mains (50 Hz): Interferes mostly with ECG and EMG
  - Radio and mobile phones
  - Diathermy (0.5–1 MHz, hence, low-pass filters used)

Pressure and its measurement

- Pressure: Force per unit area. SI unit of pressure is pascal
- Units of pressure: 1 atmosphere is equivalent to
  - 1 bar
  - 101 kPa
  - 760 mm Hg
  - 760 torr
  - 1030 cm H_2O
  - 14.6 psi (pound per square inch)

760 mm Hg = 1030 cm H_2O because mercury is denser than water.

- Gauge pressure: Pressure measured above or below the atmospheric pressure
- Absolute pressure: Pressure measured including atmospheric pressure
  - Gauge pressure + atmospheric pressure
- Manometer: U-shaped tube with fluid (water or mercury) in it. One end open to the pressure which is being measured and the other opens to a reference point
  - The reference point here is *atmospheric pressure. Hence, it is open to atmosphere*
  - Used to measure low pressures
- Barometer: U-shaped tube with fluid in it. One end open to the pressure which is being measured and the other opens to a reference point
  - The reference point here is a *vacuum. Hence it is closed at its reference point*
  - This vacuum is called the Torricellian vacuum after Evangelista Torricelli who first described its presence
- Bourdon gauge: Type of *aneroid gauge (Greek: aneroid means no water)*
  - Used to measure high pressures the manometer can't
  - Coiled metallic tube with pointer at one end and source of pressure at the other end

- o As the pressure applied to the end of the tube increases, the tube tries to straighten out
- o This then twists the pointer which will indicate a different pressure on the gauge
- Pressure regulators/pressure-reducing valves: Devices used to reduce high inlet pressures to lower outlet pressure
- Pressure in a syringe: A 2-mL syringe has a smaller cross-sectional area so the force applied by the thumb is spread over a smaller area, creating a higher pressure
  - o Area = πr^2. Hence, doubling the diameter will increase the area by a factor of 4

\# Pressure required to open an expiratory valve in an anaesthetic machine at its minimum setting is approximately 50 Pa.

Blood pressure

- Blood pressure: Pressure in blood vessels when the heart contracts or beats
  - o Invasive: Arterial line
  - o Noninvasive
    - *Continuous:* Doppler ultrasound, Penaz technique
    - *Discontinuous:* Manual cuff, automated cuff, von Recklinghausen oscillotonometer
- Invasive technique: Artery cannulated to measure blood pressure. Allen test done before cannulating radial artery
  - o Consists of arterial cannula, tubing, diaphragm (interface between fluid column and transducer), transducer (Wheatstone bridge at level of right atrium), microprocessor, amplifier and display unit. Made of Teflon
  - o Resonance: Resonance is the ability of an object to oscillate in response to a movement
    - The natural frequency of arterial transducer should be different (10 times higher) from the frequency of the arterial pressure wave or it could amplify the signal
    - Heart rate (HR) of 60/min = 1 Hz. Hence, the transducer should have a bandwidth of 0.5–40 Hz
    - Natural frequency of transducer can be increased by *short, wide cannula; short, wide tubing and stiff material.* Natural frequency is
      1. Directly related to catheter diameter
      2. Inversely related to square root of length of tubing

3. Inversely related to square root of density of fluid in the tubing

4. Inversely related to square root of system compliance

○ **Damping:** Damping is the ability of an object to resist oscillation in response to a force being applied to it

  ◆ **Overdamping:** Overdamped signals take a long time to respond to a step change. Waveform appears squashed. Underestimates systolic blood pressure (SBP), overestimates diastolic blood pressure (DBP) but *mean arterial pressure (MAP) is unaffected*

  ◆ **Underdamping:** Underdamped signals resonate around a step change. Waveform appears peaky and pointy. Overestimates SBP, underestimates DBP, but *MAP is unaffected*

  ◆ **Optimal damping:** Rapid return to zero with a minimal overshoot. *The optimal damping value is 0.64. Damping where real-time accuracy is greatest*

  ◆ **Square wave:** Used for testing clinical catheter transducer system

○ **Dicrotic notch:** Point at which aortic valve closes after the blood is ejected and is usually seen one-third of the way down the descending limb of pressure wave

  ◆ Vasodilation causes it to have a downward shift

○ *The slope of the upstroke* of arterial waveform is the best indicator of *left ventricular contractility*

○ **Position of transducer changes the MAP the most**

○ **Accuracy:** How close a measurement is to the true or accepted value

  ◆ **Precision:** How close two or more measurements are to each other, regardless of whether those measurements are accurate or not

  ◆ **Drift:** Fixed deviation from the true value at all points

• **Manual occlusive cuff method:** Cuff must cover two-thirds of the length of the limb or 20% greater than the diameter of the limb. A large cuff will underread, and *a small cuff will overread. Blood pressure is higher in legs than arms*

○ Underreads at high BPs and over reads at low BPs

○ **AF doesn't affect it while it affects the oscillotonometer.**

○ **Korotkoff method:** Auscultation over the brachial artery

  ◆ **Phase I:** *Tapping sound* – SBP is when first sound is heard

  ◆ **Phase II:** *Muffling sound* – Auscultatory gap

  ◆ **Phase III:** Reappearing of tapping sound

  ◆ **Phase IV:** Muffling sound again – DBP

  ◆ **Phase V:** Sound disappears

- **Automated occlusive cuff method:** Based on the principal of the oscillotonometer
  - Single cuff that both occludes and senses
  - As cuff is deflated, transducer detects the blood flow and the point of maximum oscillation is mean pressure
  - From the rate of change of pressure, algorithms calculate SBP and DBP
- **Von Recklinghausen's oscillotonometer:** Original machine that used two cuffs, one for occluding and another for sensing
  - Each cuff is attached to two bellows which are then attached to a single needle
  - Maximal oscillations of needle at MAP
- **Penaz technique:** Gives the continuous measurement of finger blood pressure
  - **Principle:** Force exerted on a body can be determined by measuring the opposing force that prevents physical disruption
  - The *Finapres cuff* is wrapped around the distal phalanx of a finger where it shines an infrared light which is detected on the opposite side
  - The amount of light absorbed is directly proportional to the volume of the finger
  - The volume of blood in finger keeps changing during systole and diastole
  - A *pneumatic pump* adjusts the cuff pressure to maintain a constant infrared signal
  - Pressure inside the cuff is required to achieve this displays constant blood pressure
- **Doppler ultrasound:** Based on principle of Doppler shift

Gas volume and flow measurement

- **Benedict–Roth spirometer:** Light bell is upturned into a water bath. This contains a known volume of air. This light bell is connected to a pen. The light bell moves with patient's breathing producing a spirometry trace
  - Measures gas volume rather than flow but flow can be traced
- **Vitalograph:** Single expired breath acts on bellows attached to a scribe, which marks volume on paper that moves at a constant speed
  - Vitalograph is more portable than Benedict–Roth spirometer

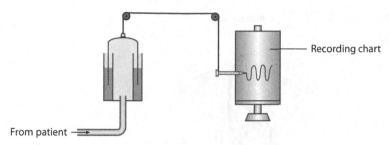

Figure 14.1 Benedict–Roth spirometer.

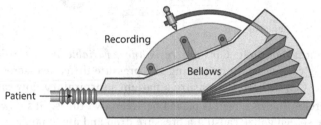

Figure 14.2 Vitalograph.

- **Wright's respirometer:** Constant pressure, variable orifice. It consists of an inlet and an outlet port. A rotating vane is present which is surrounded by slits that direct the air unidirectionally to rotate the vane
  - Used to measure tidal volume in anaesthesia
  - Placed in expiratory limb of patient
  - Accurate to 5–10%
  - Overreads at high flows
  - Underreads at low flows
  - **Water condensation can cause malfunction**

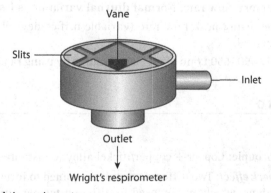

Figure 14.3 Wright's respirometer.

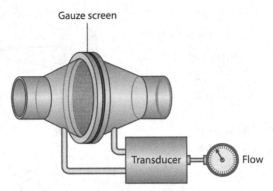

Figure 14.4   Pneumotachograph.

- **Pneumotachograph:** *Constant resistance, variable pressure flowmeter.* Flow is calculated by measuring the pressure difference across a fixed orifice. **Can be used to measure a patient's inspiratory flow rate**
    - **Screen:** Gauze screen is placed between two tubes. Gas flow through the screen gauze causing a pressure drop and any change in pressure is proportional to gas flow
    - **Fleisch:** Bundle of fine bore parallel tubes
    - **Pitot tubes:** Two pressure sampling tubes which are mounted in the centre of the gas flow
    - **Hot wire: Two hot wires mounted at right angles to each other in the lumen. Gas flows cause cooling of the wire which is then measured**
- **Rotameter: Constant pressure, variable orifice. Measures gas flow**
    - Tapered glass tube with a rotating bobbin
    - **Pressure across the bobbin remains constant and forces above and below the bobbin have equalised.**
    - In an electromagnetic flowmeter, the magnetic field is alternating as opposed to steady
- Peak expiratory flow rate: Normal diurnal variation is less than 10%
    - Measured using peak flow rate (variable orifice device). Vitalograph isn't practical
    - Normally 450–650 L/min. Can't be measured by using rapid capnograph

Temperature

A. Electrical
    - Thermocouple: Copper + copper/nickel alloy (Constantan)
        - *Seebeck effect:* Two different metals are joined to form two separate junctions, which are exposed to different temperatures producing a potential difference

- ○ **Resistance thermometer:** Electrical resistance of a pure metal increases linearly with a rise in temperature, e.g., platinum
- ○ **Thermistor: Electrical resistance in semiconductors (metal oxides) falls with a rise in temperature. Better sensitivity than resistance thermometers**

B. **Non-electrical**

- ○ **Mercury thermometer:** Solidifies at −39°C, so not used for low temperatures
- ○ **Alcohol thermometer:** Boils at 78.5°C
- ○ **Dial thermometer**
  1. Bimetallic type with two dissimilar metals with different coefficients of expansion
  2. Pressure gauge type consists of a hollow spiral metal tube

C. **Infrared:** Objects at body temperature primarily emit infrared radiation. Tympanic membrane thermometers are used

Core body temperature: Lower one-third of oesophagus, nasopharynx, tympanic, pulmonary artery flotation catheter (PAFC).

Heat loss from body

A. Radiation: *40% of heat loss* – Transfer of heat energy between two objects which are not in contact, heat loss to surroundings

B. Convection: *30% of heat loss* – Air layer adjacent to the surface of the body is warmed by convection

C. Evaporation: *25% heat loss* – Loss of latent heat of vaporisation of moisture on the skin's surface. Respiration can cause up to 10% heat loss in evaporation, 8% by humidity plus 2% warming the air

D. Conduction: *5% heat loss* – A transfer of heat from a warm object in direct contact with a cooler object

Hypothermia following induction of anaesthesia

1. **Redistribution:** Initial stage, largest drop. *Vasodilation causes heat to be shifted from core to periphery*
2. **Linear phase:** Radiation, convection, evaporation and respiration
3. **Plateau phase:** Peripheral vasoconstriction prevents further drop

Humidity

- • **Relative humidity:** Mass of water vapour in a given volume of gas as the percentage of the mass required to saturate the gas at that temperature and pressure

- **Absolute humidity:** Mass of water vapour in a given volume of gas
- **Saturated vapour pressure:** Pressure exerted by vapour phase when in equilibrium with liquid phase
- At 100% relative humidity, absolute equals
  - 17 g/m^3 at 20°C
  - 34 g/m^3 at 34°C, upper trachea
  - 44 g/m^3 at 37°C, alveoli
- Methods of measuring humidity
  - **Hair hygrometer:** Hair elongates as humidity increases. Accurate at relative humidity of 30–90%
  - **Wet and dry bulb hygrometer:** Two thermometers, one wet, one dry. The greater the humidity, the less difference there will be between the two temperatures
  - **Regnault's hygrometer:** Air blown through ether decreases temperature. Can read the temperature at which dew forms and compare it with ambient temperature using a table of saturated vapour pressures
  - Mass spectrometry
  - Ultraviolet (UV) spectroscopy
- Method to humidify inspired gases
  - Passive
    - Heat moisture exchanger (HME)
      - Hygroscopic material, conservation of latent heat
      - Expired gas warms medium, and water condenses on it
      - Inhaled gas is then warmed and humidified
      - 70–90% efficiency, 20 min to reach optimal
      - Should be changed if visibly soiled or after 48 hours
    - Cold water bubble humidifier
      - Gas bubbled through water
      - Inefficient
    - Soda lime: CO_2 production creates water
  - Active
    - Hot water bath
      - Large surface water
      - Inspired gas passes through
      - Cascade humidifier uses perforated plate to increase surface area
      - Risk of infection, electrocution and scalding

- Nebulisers (venturi or ultrasound vibration)
  - *Relative humidity can be more than 100% (oversaturation of water vapours)*
  - Large droplets (20 μm) will not travel distally

Humans acclimatize to scorching heat in a desert under a tree better than in a tropical forest because evaporation allows more heat loss in desert.

Oxygen measurement

a. Fuel (galvanic) cell
   - Anode: Lead: $Lead + OH^- \rightarrow e-$
   - Cathode: *Gold mesh:* $O_2 + 2e + H_2O \rightarrow 2OH^-$
   - Buffer: KOH
   - Current flow: pO_2
   - Reaction time: 30 s (can't be used for breath-to-breath analysis)
   - Compact and inexpensive
   - Affected by N_2O
   - Not affected by vapour
b. Clark (polarographic) electrode
   - Anode: Silver/silver chloride
   - Cathode: *Platinum*
   - Buffer: KCl/KOH
   - Small potential difference 0.6 V applied
   - Portable
c. Paramagnetic O_2 analyser
   - O_2 has *unpaired* electrons in the outer shell
   - Breath-by-breath measurement
   - Chamber: *N_2-filled chamber* with dumbbell suspended on a wire and allowed to rotate within magnetic field. *Tension of suspending ligament balances the dumbbell*
   - O_2 enters the chamber, displaces the dumbbell. Degree of rotation is proportional to concentration
   - Most commonly used in theatres. Water vapour can affect analysis
d. Mass spectrometry: Sample is continuously drawn into an apparatus. Sample is passed into an evacuated steel-ionising chamber, where it is ionised by a beam of electrons

The resulting mixture of ions then diffuse through a slit in chamber and are accelerated by a negatively charged plate. Rapid response time

Confusion buster vignette

Inhalational vapour concentration can be analysed by

- Infrared absorption (not UV radiation)
- Mass spectrometer
- Ultrasound
- Raman scattering
- Refractometer (Interferometer)
- But not paramagnetic analyser which is specific for oxygen only

Hydrogen ion and carbon dioxide measurement

- Hydrogen ion measurement: pH electrode in arterial blood gas (ABG)
  - Principle: Two solutions of different hydrogen ion concentration separated by a glass membrane develop a potential difference that is proportional to the hydrogen ion gradient between the two
  - Reading electrode (glass electrode): A silver/silver chloride electrode is enclosed in a bulb of special pH-sensitive glass and contains a buffer solution (0.1 N HCl OR KCl) that maintains a constant pH
  - Reference electrode: A silver/silver chloride electrode (previously mercury/mercury chloride) with KCl/KOH as buffer in contact with the blood via a semi-permeable membrane
  - This glass electrode is placed in the blood sample and a potential difference is generated across the glass, which is proportional to the difference in hydrogen ion concentration
  - The potential is measured between a reference electrode (in contact with the blood via a semi-permeable membrane) and the reading electrode
  - The whole system is kept at 37°C
- Carbon dioxide measurement: Done in ABG by Severinghaus electrode and in anaesthetic machine by capnography, colorimetry, Raman spectroscopy and mass spectroscopy (discussed in chapter 'Capnography')
  - Severinghaus or CO_2 electrode
    - Principle: Carbon dioxide, but not hydrogen ions, diffuses from the blood sample across the membrane into the sodium bicarbonate solution, producing hydrogen ions and a change in pH

- **Reading electrode (Severinghaus electrode):** A modified pH electrode (Ag/AgCl in KCl buffer solution with glass tip) in contact with sodium bicarbonate solution and separated from the blood specimen by a rubber or Teflon semi-permeable membrane
- **Reference electrode:** A silver/silver chloride electrode (previously mercury/mercury chloride) with KCl/KOH as buffer in contact with the blood via a semi-permeable membrane
- Slow response time due to diffusion of CO_2 across the Teflon membrane
- **pH stat and alpha stat: Solubility of gases in a solution increases with fall in temperature**
   - Analysis of a sample taken from a hypothermic patient occurs at 37°C. The pO_2 and pCO_2 results are artificially high because they come out in blood with heating up of solution
   - Cooling of a solution causes the pH of solution to increase
   - Cardiac anaesthetists face this dilemma while reading the ABG of patients on deep hypothermic cardiac arrest
   - **pH stat approach:** $PaCO_2$ is maintained at 40 mm Hg and the pH is maintained at 7.40 when measured at the patient's actual low temperature, i.e., hypothermia
      - Therefore, CO_2 is added to the inspired gas via the oxygenator to negate the increased solubility of CO_2 at lower temperatures
   - Alpha stat approach: $PaCO_2$ and the pH are maintained at 40 mm Hg and 7.40 when measured at 37°C, i.e., the blood sample is warmed to normothermia for measurement

Cardiac output monitoring

- **Cardiac output (CO):** Volume of blood ejected by each ventricle per minute. CO = stroke volume (SV) × HR
   - Thermodilution method using pulmonary artery catheter (PAC) is still considered the gold standard method
- **Thermodilution method:** Injection and sampling are carried out via a catheter in the right side of the heart
   - Cold fluid is injected into the right atrium and the temperature change is detected by a thermistor at the distal end of the PAC
   - A temperature change against time curve is generated and CO is estimated as its inversely related to the area under the curve (AUC)
   - Dye (indocyanine green) or indicator (lithium) use the same principle, but the sampling for them happens in a peripheral arterial blood sample

- **Fick's principle:** The uptake or excretion of a substance by an organ or tissue must be equal to the difference between the amount entering or leaving the organ
  - $DO_2 = CO \times (CaO_2 - CvO_2)$

    where DO_2 is oxygen uptake, CO is cardiac output, CaO_2 is arterial oxygen content, CvO_2 is mixed venous oxygen content (PAC)
  - Oxygen uptake is measured via spirometry
- **Oesophageal Doppler:** The shift in frequency is proportional to the velocity of ejected blood
  - The device generates a velocity/time waveform which is calibrated using patient's height, weight and age. **Probe inserted reaching 40 cm**
  - SV is then derived from flow velocity ejection time and aortic area
  - Measures flow in **descending thoracic aorta** which is 70% of total flow
  - Corrected systolic flow time (FT_c) is generated which is normally between 330 and 360 ms and a low FT_c indicates inadequate volume in vessels
- **Arterial pulse contour:** Based on the principle that area under the systolic part of the arterial pressure waveform is proportional to the SV
  - CO is proportional to arterial pulse pressure
  - PiCCO: Calibrated via transpulmonary thermodilution technique
    - Central venous catheter (CVC) and a central artery catheter (femoral)
    - Provides stroke volume variation (SVV), pulse pressure variation (PPV), systolic pressure variation (SPV)
  - LiDCO: Calibrated via lithium dilution technique
    - CVC and a peripheral artery catheter (radial)
    - Provides SVV, PPV and SPV

\# Area under arterial trace is the best reflection of CO.

- **Transthoracic electrical bioimpedance:** Based on the principle that during systole, ejection of blood from the heart is associated with change in electrical impedance of the thoracic cavity due to increased blood volume
  - Rate of change of this impedance is proportional to CO
  - Four electrodes are placed on the neck and thorax and a low current is passed between them

- o Blood volume and velocity within the aorta changes from beat to beat and this leads to changes in thoracic impedance
- o Device measures the changes in impedance and signifies CO

Peripheral nerve stimulators

- Two types of peripheral nerve stimulators
  - o Assess degree of neuromuscular blockade
  - o Aid nerve blockade for regional anaesthesia
- Assess degree of neuromuscular blockade
  - o Mechanomyography: Measures the isometric contraction force in the adductor pollicis after ulnar nerve stimulation. Used for research
  - o Acceleromyography: Small piezoelectric transducer to measure the isotonic acceleration of the muscle. Used for research
  - o EMG: Measures electrical activity of the stimulated muscle just prior to contraction. Used for research
  - o Clinical signs: Ability to keep head lifted for 5 s, hand grip strength. Crude methods
  - o Nerve stimulation: All twitches are given at supramaximal current stimulus 50 mA. All twitches last just 0.2 ms
    - *Single twitch*: Single stimulus at frequency of 1 Hz
    - *Train of four (TOF)*: Four stimulus at frequency of 2 Hz. Fade is seen
      - – 1–2 twitches seen: Surgery can be done
      - – 3–4 twitches seen: Attempt reversal
    - *Tetanic stimulation*: 250 stimuli over a duration of 5 s at a frequency of 50 Hz
    - *Post-tetanic count (PTC)*: Stimulus given after a tetanic stimulation. Used for deep degree of neuromuscular blockade. Frequency is 1 Hz
      - – PTC <5 = Profound block
      - – PTC >5 = Two twitches on TOF
    - *Double burst stimulation (DBS)*: Three twitches at frequency of 50 Hz followed by a break of 750 ms and then another three twitches at frequency of 50 Hz

DBS is the most sensitive way to test incomplete reversal.

- Aid nerve blockade for regional anaesthesia
  - Current strength used: 0.1–1 mA
  - Current is applied to the needle at low amplitude that is 1 mA to locate nerve. As needle gets closer to nerve, current is reduced to 0.2–0.3 mA before giving local anaesthetic
- **Fade:** Phenomenon of decreasing twitch height after repetitive stimuluses are given post–administration of neuromuscular blocking drugs
- **Post-tetanic potentiation:** Tetanic stimulation is sufficient to produce a substantial increase in acetylcholine release to overcome competition from neuromuscular blocking drugs most of the time
- **Phase I block:** Seen after single dose of suxamethonium
  - Fade and post-tetanic facilitation is not seen
  - May be potentiated by anticholinesterases, volatile agents, magnesium and lithium
  - Dantrolene doesn't antagonise it
- **Phase II block:** Seen after repeated doses of suxamethonium
  - Exhibits fade and post-tetanic facilitation
- **Diaphragm is most resistant muscle of all** and requires twice the dose for the same effect as the muscle normally used for twitches, which is the adductor pollicis (ulnar nerve). Other nerves that can be used for twitches are facial (orbicularis oculi) and posterior tibial nerve (flexor hallucis brevis)
- **Adequate reversal if TOF > 0.9**

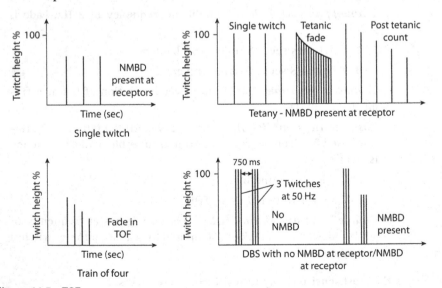

Figure 14.5   TOF.

Depth of anaesthesia monitoring

- **Clinical signs:** High blood pressure, tachycardia, sweating and tear formation are used by anaesthetists to measure depth of anaesthesia measurement
- **Isolated forearm technique:** A pneumatic cuff is wrapped around the patient's upper arm and inflated above systolic pressure
  - A neuromuscular blocking agent is given after this; hence, the lower arm is not paralysed
  - Thus, the patient, if aware, can squeeze the anaesthetist's hand
- **Raw EEG interpretation:** EEG electrodes are positioned on the patient's head to record the characteristic potentials arising from the activity of the cortex
  - Increase in depth of anaesthesia is associated with a decrease in the frequency and amplitude of the EEG
  - Burst suppression of the EEG occurs at a deep level of anaesthesia
- **Bispectral Index (BIS):** A four-electrode sensor is placed on the patient's forehead. A proprietary algorithm processes the EEG data
  - Shows similar changes with most anaesthetic agents except ketamine
  - Can't predict response to surgical incision
  - Can't differentiate between ischaemia and sedation, falls with both
    - 0–20: Burst suppression
    - 20–40: Deep hypnosis
    - 40–60: Surgical anaesthesia
    - 60–80: Arousable with stimulation
    - 80–100: Awake and explicit recall
- **E-entropy monitor:** Three electrode sensor placed on the patient's forehead. It measures the irregularity in spontaneous brain (EEG) and facial muscular activity (EMG)
  - EEG and EMG activity produce two numbers response entropy (RE) and state entropy (SE)
  - RE range is 0–100 (awake) and SE range is 0–91. Target range is 40–60
- **Narco-trend:** Pattern recognition of the raw EEG and classifies the EEG epochs
  - Six-letter classification from A (awake) to F (general anaesthesia with increasing burst suppression)
  - Divided into 14 substages (A, B: 0–2, C: 0–2, D: 0–2, E: 0,1; F: 0,1)

- **Auditory-evoked potential (AEP):** Auditory sense disappears when undergoing anaesthesia
  - A number of clicks are delivered to the patient's ear once they are anaesthetised
  - EEG is monitored and analysed to give an AEP index
  - AEP >80 is awake, AEP <50 is asleep

Cerebral monitoring

- Intracranial pressure monitoring
  - **External ventricular drain (EVD):** Gold standard. Allows both cerebrospinal fluid (CSF) measurement and drainage of CSF
  - **Epidural bolt:** Most commonly used device. Fibreoptic probe inserted between dura and skull via a burr hole
  - **Subarachnoid bolt:** Relatively easy to install via burr hole but high infection rates
- Cerebral oxygenation
  - **Jugular venous oxygen saturation:** Global assessment of oxygenation
    - A catheter is inserted by retrograde cannulation of the internal jugular vein and advanced into the jugular bulb
    - Fibreoptic catheter similar to monitoring of mixed venous oxygen saturation in the pulmonary artery is used for continuous $SjVO_2$ monitoring
    - Dominant side of brain, mostly right-sided cannulation
    - Normal $SjvO_2$ is 55–75%
    - Used in severe traumatic brain injury (TBI) to guide interventions like hyperventilation
  - **Near-infrared spectroscopy:** Regional assessment of oxygenation. Non-invasive
    - Near-infrared light (700–1000 nm) is shone through the layers of the brain. The light is reflected and absorbed by different tissues with absorption dependent upon the oxygenation status
    - Beer–Lambert law is used
    - Normal regional oxygen saturation (rSO_2) is 60–75%
    - Used in cardiac surgery and carotid endarterectomy
- Cerebral blood flow monitoring
  - **Transcranial Doppler:** Non-invasive
    - Doppler effect is where the observed frequency of a signal increases as the source moves towards the observer

* The velocity of blood flow is directly related to the change in transmitted frequency of a sound wave
* Flow velocities can be measured in the intracranial arteries
* Used mainly to monitor for vasospasm after subarachnoid haemorrhage
* Can detect microemboli as well

Thromboelastography

* **Thromboelastography (TEG):** Point of care test which helps to identify specific factors that may be inhibiting the process of clot formation
* **Principle:** A cup containing a sample of blood which is placed in the machine. A torsion wire is suspended within the sample. Cup is rotated and the wire becomes linked by the sample. A torsional force is therefore applied to the wire. As the clot becomes stronger, amplitude of TEG trace increases
* **Parameters**
  * **R-value (Reaction time):** Time taken from beginning of test until initial clot formation
    * **Normal value:** 20–30 mm or 5–10 min
    * Increased by factor deficiency or heparinisation
    * Treated by fresh frozen plasma (FFP)
  * **K-value (clot kinetics):** Time taken to achieve a clot strength of 20-mm amplitude
    * **Normal value:** 8–15 mm or 1–5 min
    * Increased by fibrinogen deficiency
    * Treated by cryoprecipitate
  * **α angle (reaction time):** Angle between R + 1 mm and K. Rate at which fibrin cross-linking occurs
    * **Normal value:** 60–75°
    * Decreased by **fibrinogen deficiency**
    * **Treated by cryoprecipitate**
  * **Maximum amplitude (MA):** Measure of clot strength. Maximum point is taken
    * **Normal value:** 50–75 mm
    * Decreased by platelet deficiency or platelet function
    * Treated by platelets

- o LY-30 (clot lysis): Degradation of clot 30 min after MA is achieved
  - ◆ Normal value: 0–10%
  - ◆ Increased by increased clot breakdown
  - ◆ Treated by tranexamic acid
- Sensitive to heparin, although any heparin effect can be blocked by adding heparinase to blood sample. Heparinised sample: Flat line

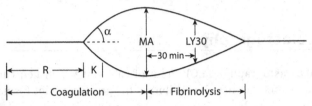

Figure 14.6   TEG.

Anaesthesia Equipment

15

Medical gases

- Oxygen: Commercial oxygen (99% pure) is produced by fractional distillation of liquefied air. Oxygen concentrators use zeolite adsorbers to produce O_2 that is 90–93% pure (argon is main contaminant) and are used for portable oxygen production like in military field or home
  - Stored in vacuum-insulated evaporator (VIE)
    - VIE has an inner stainless-steel tank with outer steel jacket
    - Holds up 1500 L of 'liquid' oxygen between −160 and −180°C
    - Oxygen is stored at 1000 kPa with a safety valve that blows up at 1500 kPa
    - A gauge indicates the pressure within, and a differential pressure gauge (compares top to bottom) indicates the oxygen contents by weight
  - Hospital backup oxygen supply is from size J cylinders arranged in series (cylinder manifold)
  - Cylinders used in anaesthetic machines are made up of molybdenum steel and are size E
- Nitrous oxide: Produced by heating ammonium nitrate at 240°C
  - $NH_4NO_3 \rightarrow N_2O + 2H_2O$. Impurities like NH_3, N_2, NO_2 are removed prior to storage
  - Storage of nitrous oxide is done in a central bank of gas cylinders
- Medical air: Generated by compressing atmospheric air. Contains oil and water vapour as impurities
  - Low-pressure supply (420 kPa): Anaesthetic machines and ventilators
  - Higher-pressure supply (700 kPa): Power for surgical equipment
- Xenon: Produced by fractional distillation of liquefied air. Stored in a gas in cylinder at room temperature above 16°C, which is the critical temperature of xenon
- Entonox: Produced by blending 50% N_2O with 50% O_2. Stored in cylinders

DOI: 10.1201/9781003390244-18

- **Carbon dioxide:** This is a waste product of manufacturing processes. Gaseous CO_2 is collected, filtered, dried, compressed and liquefied. It is then stored as a liquid in cylinders
- **Definitions**
  - ○ **Gas:** Molecule above its critical temperature
  - ○ **Vapour:** Molecule below its critical temperature
  - ○ **Critical temperature:** Temperature above which a molecule cannot be liquified no matter how much pressure is used
  - ○ **Critical pressure:** Pressure required to liquefy a gas at its critical temperature
  - ○ **Pseudocritical temperature:** Temperature at which gases separate into their individual constituents, e.g., –7°C for Entonox cylinder
  - ○ **Poynting effect:** O_2, when bubbled through liquid N_2O, forms a gaseous O_2/N_2O mixture. This effect is known as the Poynting effect

Gas cylinders

Molecule	Gas or vapour	Cylinder Pressure (bar)	Critical temperature (°C)	Colour coding Cylinder	Colour coding Shoulder	Pin index
Oxygen	Gas	137	–119	Black	White	2,5
Air	Gas	137		Black	White/ black	1,5
Nitrous oxide	**Vapour**	44	36.5	Blue	Blue	3,5
Carbon dioxide	Vapour	50	31	Grey	Grey	1,6 (>7.5%) 2,6 (<7.5%)
Entonox	Gas/ vapour mix	137		Blue	Blue/ white	7
Helium	Gas	137	–268	Brown	Brown	No pin

- Medical cylinders are made up of **molybdenum steel**
- Cylinder markings/labels
  - ○ Serial number of cylinder
  - ○ Symbol of gas

- o Density of gas
- o Hydraulic test pressure of cylinder
- o **Tare weight of cylinder:** Weight of empty cylinder
  - • **E cylinder:** *Anaesthetic machine* – water capacity of 4.7 L
  - • **J cylinder:** *Storage* – water capacity of 47 L
- Cylinders are tested for safety every 5–10 years
  - o Endoscopic examination
  - o **Tensile tests:** 1% of cylinders are destroyed to perform testing on the metal
- The **filling ratio** is the weight of liquid in a full cylinder compared with the weight of water that would completely fill the cylinder
  - o In cool climates, the filling ratio is 0.75
  - o In warmer climates, the filling ratio is reduced to 0.67
- The **pin index system:** Used to prevent the wrong gas yoke being connected to a cylinder
  - o Pins protrude from the back of the yoke on the anaesthetic machine
  - o Holes exist on the valve block of the cylinder
  - o Pins and holes must line up for the cylinder to be connected
- **Critical temperature:** Temperature above which a substance cannot be liquefied no matter what pressure is applied
- **Critical pressure:** *Pressure required to liquefy gas at its critical temperature*
  - o It is pressure above which a liquid cannot be boiled

Entonox has a two-stage valve to allow on-demand delivery when a negative pressure is developed in the second-stage valve.

Breathing circuits

- **Breathing systems:** System used to deliver fresh gases and volatile agents to patient
- Classified into open and closed systems
  - o **Open system:** Oxygen mask
  - o **Closed system:** Classified into rebreathing and non-rebreathing systems
    - • **Rebreathing system:** Mapleson circuits
    - • **Non-rebreathing system:** Circle system

Mapleson classification	Spontaneous ventilation	Controlled ventilation	Comments
A (Magill)	70 mL/kg/min	2–3 MV	- Good for spontaneous ventilation - 'Lack' system is a coaxial system
B	2–3 MV	2–3 MV	- Not used
C (Waters)	2–3 MV	2–3 MV	- Used for resuscitation or transfer
D	2–3 MV	- 70 mL/kg/min or 2–3 MV - **Bain:** Inner tube carries fresh gas flow	- Good for controlled ventilation - 'Bain' circuit is coaxial system. Can be used in children <20 kg
E (Ayre's T-piece)	2–3 MV	2–3 MV	- Suitable for paediatrics
F (Jackson–Rees modification of Ayre's T-piece)	2–3 MV	2–3 MV	- Suitable for paediatrics (occupational hazard for anaesthetists though)

In Bains circuit, if a patient's fresh gas flow (FGF) is greater than minute ventilation (MV) and the reservoir bag falls down, nothing will happen as FGF is greater than MV.

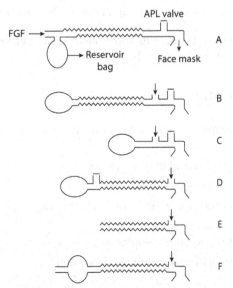

Figure 15.1 Mapleson circuits.

Anaesthesia machine

- Safety features in anaesthesia machine
  - Gas supplies
    - Pipelines: *4.1 bar*
      1. Colour-coded flexible hosepipes
      2. *Schrader valve* connects hosepipes to wall (gas specific and non-interchangeable due to varying sizes of collar on probes)
         - Each specific gas probe has a particular collar size to open the matching valve on the Schrader outlet
      3. *Non-interchangeable screw threads (NIST)* connect hosepipes to anaesthetic machine (gas-specific and permanently fixed)
    - Cylinders
      1. Colour-coded gas cylinders
      2. Pin-indexed system
      3. Symbol of gas
      4. Cylinder labels
      5. Safety relief device (frangible disc or fusible plug or safety relieve valve)
  - Flowmeters: Reduce pressure from 4 bar to just above atmospheric pressure
    - Oxygen is the last gas to be added to the FGF
    - Oxygen control knob is labelled and colour coded
    - Oxygen control knob is larger and protrudes out
    - Anti-static spray in flowmeter
    - **Mandatory minimum oxygen flow: 150–250 mL/min**
  - **Hypoxia prevention safety devices**
    - **Link 25 proportioning system (Datex Ohmeda):** 14-tooth sprocket (N_2O) and 28-tooth sprocket (O_2). Minimum oxygen concentration of 25%
    - **Sensitive oxygen ratio controller (S-ORC) (Drager):** Fail-safe component shuts off nitrous oxide if the oxygen flow is less than 200 mL/min
  - **Oxygen failure warning device**
    - Activated when the oxygen supply pressure falls below 2 bar, alarm of 60 dB for a minimum of 7 s
  - **Oxygen flush**
    - 100% oxygen is supplied at 40–70 L/min

- o Vaporisers
  - ◆ Colour-coded vaporisers
  - ◆ Filling devices are geometrically coded and agent specific
  - ◆ **Interlock system:** Prevents more than one vaporiser being used at the same time
  - ◆ Unidirectional check valve
  - ◆ Back pressure relief valve
- o **Common gas outlet**
  - ◆ Standardised 22-mm male outer diameter/15-mm female internal diameter
- o **Breathing system**
  - ◆ Adjustable pressure-limiting (APL) valve opens if pressure exceeds above 70 cm H_2O
- o **Scavenging**
  - ◆ Throws hazardous gases outside the theatre complex
- o **Monitoring**
  - ◆ Oxygen, CO_2 and inhalational agents are essential and displayed continuously

 # Volumetric pumps: Employ a linear peristaltic pumping mechanism or use a special cassette. They have a specific delivery, e.g., epidural pump.

Vaporisers

- **Vapour:** A substance in the gaseous phase, below its critical temperature
- **Vapour pressure:** The proportion of atmospheric pressure, i.e., partial pressure attributable to a vapour
- **Saturated vapour pressure:** The partial pressure generated by a vapour in equilibrium with its liquid form at standard temperature and pressure (STP)
  - o The partial pressure and, hence, standard vapour pressure (SVP) of a gas agent depends only on the temperature of the liquid
- **Boiling point:** A liquid boils when the saturated vapour pressure equals ambient pressure
  - o At lower ambient pressures, liquid boils at lower temperatures
- **Classification of vaporisers:** The purpose of a vaporiser is to reliably deliver an accurate, adjustable concentration of anaesthetic vapour
  - o **Variable bypass vaporisers:** Having an adjustable proportion of gas that either enters or bypasses a vaporising chamber
    - ◆ **Plenum vaporisers:** High internal resistance requiring fresh gas is greater than atmospheric pressure. e.g., Tec 5 and Tec 7

- **Draw over vaporisers:** FGF at atmospheric pressure, driven by the patient's respiratory efforts. Must have a non-rebreathing valve. Oxford miniature vaporiser
- ○ **Measured flow vaporisers:** By adding vapour directly to the FGF, e.g., desflurane Tec 6
- **Plenum vaporisers:** Objective is to deliver the same concentration of anaesthetic agent over a range of flows. They do so by adjusting gas flow rates and temperature as mentioned
  - ○ **Gas flow rates:** As the FGF rate increases, it becomes more difficult to achieve full saturation of gas leaving the vaporising chamber
    - *Wicks:* These increase the surface area from which the gas has to 'pick up' vapour, making it easier to maintain concentration with high flow rates
    - *Baffles:* These make the FGF come in repeated contact with the vaporising surface, increasing the uptake of agent and ensuring a constant uptake with high flows
    - *Bubbles:* Bubbling the FGF through the anaesthetic agent increases the surface area for uptake making it easier to keep constant concentrations with high flow rates
  - ○ **Temperature:** The SVP of an agent and, hence, the vaporiser output decreases nonlinearly with decreasing temperature. The methods to stabilize it are
    - **Temperature stabilisation:** Making the vaporiser with materials with high specific heat capacity and thermal conductivity provides a heat sink, allowing heat to move rapidly between the vaporising chamber and the atmosphere
    - **Temperature compensation:** Devices that changes the splitting ratio when the temperature changes
      1. *Bimetallic strip:* Bimetallic strips are strips made of two metals, each of which expand at different rates when the temperature rises. This causes the tip of the strip to move, opening up the entrance of the vaporising chamber. They are major method of temperature compensation
      2. *Aneroid bellows:* These are connected by a rod to a cone in the orifice of the bypass chamber. A reduction in temperature causes the bellows to contract, resulting in the cone partially obstructing the bypass channel, increasing flow through the vaporising chamber
  - ○ **Pumping effect:** Pressure from gas-driven ventilators is transmitted in a retrograde fashion to the back bar and vaporiser. Saturated gas can be forced back through the vaporiser inlet port and enter the bypass channel resulting in increased agent delivery

♦ A one-way valve at the outflow of the vaporiser ensures that the vaporising chamber and bypass chamber are of equal volumes so backpressure is transmitted equally to both or that the vaporiser inflow port is long
- Measured flow vaporisers: They have a separate stream of agent-saturated gas that is added to the gas flow
  - Tec 6 vaporiser: Desflurane is very volatile and has a boiling point of 23°C. Small changes in ambient temperature would result in large changes in desflurane's SVP
    ♦ The desflurane vaporiser heats the anaesthetic agent to 39°C to ensure a constant SVP
    ♦ This anaesthetic vapour is injected into the FGF downstream the vasporisation chamber

Scavenging system

- Adverse effects of volatile agents and N$_2$O
  - Global warming
  - Damage in the ozone layer
  - N$_2$O can cause bone marrow toxicity and peripheral neuropathy
  - Spontaneous miscarriages
  - Infertility
- Scavenging: Scavenging is the collection and removal of vented anaesthetic gases from the operation theatre
- Active scavenging system
  - Collection system: Shroud that connects with APL valve by a 30-mm connector
  - Transfer system: Wide boring tube
  - Receiving system: Reservoir with visual flow indicator
  - Disposal system: Air pump creates a vacuum and throws the waste to outside atmosphere
- Passive scavenging system
  - No external power or vacuum used
  - Patient's spontaneous respiratory efforts throw out gases
  - Cardiff Aldasorber: Passive type of system with cannister containing charcoal particles that absorb halogenated volatile anaesthetic agents
- Control of substances hazardous to health (COSHH): Sets safe maximum exposure limits to chemicals and other hazardous substances

- Theatre ventilation should ensure 15 air changes per hour
- Maximum recommended anaesthetic pollutant levels based on an 8-hour time-weighted average (TWA)
  - Halothane: 10 parts per million (ppm)
  - Isoflurane: 50 ppm
  - Nitrous oxide: 100 ppm

Soda lime

- Soda lime: Absorbs CO_2. 80% Ca $(OH)_2$ + 2% NaOH + 16% H_2O
  - Phenolphthalein is a dye that changes colour from pink to white, ethyl violet changes colour from white to purple. **So colour changes depend upon dye**
  - Silicates are added in trace amounts to harden the granules
  - **Soda lime if left unused can regenerate**
  - The granule size is between 4 and 8 mesh. (Mesh is the number of openings per inch in a uniform metal strainer or they will pass through a mesh with four to eight strands per inch in each axis)
  - Reaction is
    - $CO_2 + H_2O \rightarrow H_2CO_3$
    - $H_2CO_3 + 2NaOH \rightarrow Na_2CO_3 + 2H_2O + Heat$
    - Ca $(OH)_2 + Na_2CO_3 \rightarrow CaCO_3 + 2NaOH + Heat$
    - Overall, $CO_2 + Ca (OH)_2 \rightarrow CaCO_3 + H_2O$
    - **So, water increases absorption of CO_2**
  - **Soda lime reacts with sevoflurane to form compound A.** Hepatotoxicity, renal toxicity and brain damage in rats; however, no evidence of such effects in humans
  - **Dry soda lime reacts with desflurane, isoflurane and enflurane (CHF_2 containing agents) to produce carbon monoxide**
  - **KOH was previously in this** but was implicated with a higher tendency to form carbon monoxide and compound A, so it was removed
- **Baralyme/Barium lime: 80% Ca $(OH)_2$ + 20% Ba (OH_2). Barium hydroxide already has H_2O**
  - Less efficient than soda lime
  - Reaction with sevoflurane is five times faster
- **Amsorb: Ca $(OH)_2$ + $CaCl_2$**
  - Not associated with compound A or carbon monoxide formation

Ventilators

- **Mechanical ventilators:** Automatically inflates the lungs when the patient is unable to breathe spontaneously
  - **Negative pressure ventilation:** Iron lung
  - **Positive pressure ventilation:** Current ventilators

Method of classification	Classification	Process
Cycling method (Change over from inspiration to exhalation and vice versa)	Volume cycling	When the predetermined tidal volume is reached during inspiration, the ventilator changes to exhalation
	Pressure cycling	Stiffer the lung, quicker the pressure is achieved
	Time cycling	Using mechanical, pneumatic or electronic timers. Most commonly used method
	Volume cycling	Older ventilators
Method of operation	Flow generator	- Ventilator produces inspiration by generating a constant and predetermined pressure - Can't compensate for leaks in the system - Can compensate for changes in lung compliance
	Pressure generator	- Ventilator produces inspiration by delivering a predetermined flow of gas - Can compensate for leaks in the system - Can't compensate for changes in lung compliance
Source of power	Pneumatic	Uses compressed gas as its power source
	Electrical	Electrically powered
	Combined	Pneumatically powered but electronically controlled
Place of use	Intensive care unit (ICU)	Used mostly for ICU patients
	Operating theatres (OTs)	Used mainly for operating theatres

(*Continued*)

Method of classification	Classification	Process
Paediatric use	Yes/No	Suitable for children
Special features	SIMV, PS, PEEP	Availability of newer modes
Function	Mechanical thumbs	- Pressurised gas connected to a T-piece and thumb/valve used to occlude one end and give intermittent ventilation. Neonatal anaesthesia
	Minute volume dividers	- Fresh gas flow is equal to minute ventilation and is stored in a reservoir and delivered in divided tidal volumes
	Bottle in bag	- Bellows in a chamber. Electronically powered
	Lightweight portable	- Powered by compressed gas (intermittent blower)

- **Manley MP3 ventilator:** Ventilator invented around the 1960s
  - Pneumatically powered, time-cycled, MV divider
  - Required no external power source, was connected to the fresh gas outlet of the anaesthetic machine and delivered the gas to the patient as an MV divider
  - All the FGF (the MV) is delivered to the patient divided into readily set tidal volumes
  - FGF fills a series of bellows, and a sliding weight provides pressure to inflate lungs
  - Consists of two sets of bellows, three unidirectional valves, an APL valve and a reservoir bag
- **Servo 900 series ventilator**
  - Pneumatically driven, electronically controlled, MV divider
  - A bellows bag is filled with FGF but a spring instead of FGF compresses the bag to push FGF into the inspiratory limb. Therefore, this is not a bag-in-bottle system
  - Expiratory limb is vented to scavenging; hence, not a circle breathing system

- **Penlon–Nuffield:** Intermittent blower ventilators driven by a high pressure (400 kPa). They are constant flow generators
  - Pneumatically powered, time-cycled, intermittent blower
  - Inspiratory and expiratory time and flow controls
  - Addition of Newton valve makes it a time-cycled, pressure generator; hence, it can be used in children
- **Oxylog 3000:** Used for transport of patients
  - Pneumatically powered, electronically controlled, time-cycled, intermittent blower
- **Bag-in-bottle ventilator:** Bellows inside a chamber like in modern ventilators such as the Ohmeda anaesthetic machine ventilator
  - Pneumatically powered, electronically controlled, time-cycled, bag squeezer
  - Compressed air is used as the driving gas. On entering the chamber, the compressed air forces the bellows (containing FGF) down, delivering the fresh gas to the patient

Cleaning and sterilisation

- **Cleaning:** Physical removal of foreign material from equipment without destroying infectious agents. It lowers the bioburden before it is subjected to disinfection or sterilisation
- **Disinfection:** Elimination of all pathogenic organisms except bacterial spores. Chemicals used to disinfect inanimate physical objects are known as *disinfectants*. Chemicals used to disinfect human body surfaces are known as *antiseptics*
  - **High-level disinfection:** All bacteria except endospores, fungi and viruses
  - **Low-level disinfection:** All bacteria except tuberculosis (TB) and endospores, some fungi, some viruses
- **Sterilisation:** Elimination of all pathogenic organisms except bacterial spores
- **Spaulding classification**
  - **Critical:** Items that enter sterile tissue or the vascular system of body, e.g., surgical instruments, needles. Items should be sterilised
  - **Semi-critical:** Items that contact mucous membranes and non-intact skin but do not break the blood barrier, e.g., laryngoscopes, endoscopes. Sterilisation or high-level disinfection
  - **Non-critical:** Items that come into contact with healthy skin but not mucous membranes, e.g., pulse-oximeter. Low-level disinfection or cleaning

Method	Technique	Procedure		Used for
Cleaning	Manual	Cold water washing		Blood pressure (BP) cuffs/stethoscopes
	Automated	Ultrasonic baths		
Disinfection	Chemical	High-level disinfection	Glutaraldehyde (1–1.5%)	Endoscope
			Hydrogen peroxide	Fogging of operating theatre
			Peracetic acid	Fibrescope
		Low-level disinfection	Alcohol	Alcohol based rubs
			Sodium hypochlorite	Surface disinfectants/ blood spills
	Heat (Pasteurisation)	20 min at 70°C		Semi-critical items like breathing tubes, face masks
Sterilisation	Steam	Dry heat: 150 for 30 minutes		Glassware
		Moist heat (autoclave): 122°C for 30 min at 1 atm or 134°C for 3 min at 2 atm		Metal items like forceps
	Chemical	Ethylene oxide		Heat labile items but can be toxic
	Gas plasma	Ionised gas		Heat labile items but non-toxic
	Radiation	Gamma rays from cobalt-60		Heat labile sharps

Pulse oximetry

- Pulse oximetry: Equipment used to measure the percentage of haemoglobin saturated with oxygen in arterial blood
- Principle: *Beer–Lambert law* – The law states that the absorbance of a solution depends on
  - Lambert: The path length of light travelling through the solution
  - Beer: The concentration of that solution
  - Absorbance (A) = $\varepsilon l c$
    - A is absorbance of the solution
    - ε = Molar absorption coefficient
    - l = Length of solution that the light passes through
    - c = Concentration of the compound in solution in mol/L

- o Absorption from arterial blood is pulsatile, whereas the signal from venous haemoglobin and tissue is not. When the arteries pulsate, the distance travelled by light though them changes **(Lambert)**
- o Concentration of oxyhaemoglobin and deoxyhaemoglobin can be determined from their absorption of the two wavelengths **(Beer)**
- **Equipment:** Two light-emitting diodes (LEDs) and a photodiode. Light from LEDs blinks and goes through the patient and is detected by the photodiode
  - o One LED emits at **660 nm (red)** and the other at **940 nm (infrared)**
  - o Oxyhaemoglobin absorbs more infrared (940 nm) and emits red light (660 nm)
  - o Deoxyhaemoglobin absorbs more red light and emits infrared to pass through
  - o LEDs flash in sequence one after another and then both go off to allow for correction for ambient light
  - o The microprocessor corrects for ambient light and for the difference between the arterial and venous saturations
  - o Isosbestic point: The absorption of deoxyhaemoglobin and oxyhae-moglobin is the same at 805nm, which is known as the isosbestic point
  - o Analysis of the absorption of infrared at 805nm allows quantification of the total concentration of haemoglobin present
  - o Haemoglobin saturation = $\dfrac{HbO_2 \times 100\%}{Hb + HbO_2}$

  where HbO_2 is concentration of oxyhaemoglobin measured at 660 nm and Hb is concentration of deoxyhaemoglobin measured at 940 nm
- **Source of errors**
  - o **Low perfusion states (hypotension):** Shows saturation at 85%
  - o **Methaemoglobin:** Shows saturation at 85%
  - o **Dyes like methylene blue/disulphine blue/indocyanine green:** Abnormally low readings
  - o **Carboxyhaemoglobin (HbCO):** High saturation readings despite low oxyhaemoglobin
  - o **Cyanide poison:** High saturation readings despite low oxyhaemoglobin
  - o **HbS/HbF/sulfhaemoglobin:** No effect on oximetry
  - o **Skin pigmentation** has no effect on oximetry
- **Pulse oximeters have a faster response time than transcutaneous oxygen electrodes**

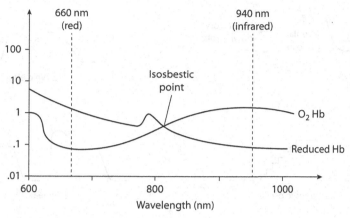

Figure 15.2 Pulse oximeter principle.

Capnography

- **Capnography:** Continuous measurement and pictorial display of end-tidal CO_2
  - ○ **Capnometry:** Only measurement of end-tidal CO_2
  - ○ **Capnogram:** Pictorial trace showing end-tidal CO_2
- **Principle:** *Infrared absorption* – Most commonly used monitor
  - ○ A molecule with two different atoms (diatomic) will absorb infrared radiation, e.g., CO_2 and N_2O
  - ○ For CO_2, the absorption is maximal at 4.28 μm
  - ○ A hot wire emits infrared radiation. This beam is split between reference and sample gas chambers
  - ○ Windows of both reference and sample gas chambers are made of sapphire as glass absorbs infrared radiation
  - ○ By measuring the proportion of infrared radiation absorbed by CO_2, its partial pressure can be measured
  - ○ Water vapours are trapped inside as they have high infrared absorbance
  - ○ **Collision broadening:** Broadening of the bandwidth of infrared absorption of carbon dioxide due to presence of N_2O molecules around
  - ○ **Side stream capnography sampling tube is made of Teflon.** Sampling at 150 mL/min. Sampling tube length is 2 m
- **Colourimetry:** Carbon dioxide will react with water to form carbonic acid which will change the pH. This will change the colour of the indicator. Used in portable devices intended to confirm correct tracheal tube placement

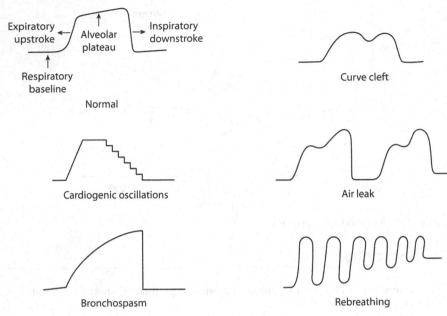

Figure 15.3   Capnographs.

- **Mass spectrometry:** Gas sample is introduced into an ionisation chamber. These gas molecules are bombarded by a beam of electrons. Some of the gas molecules can become charged and are then deflected by another charged plate according to their mass
  - Accurate and very rapid response time (can create capnograph)
  - Bulky and very large
- **Raman spectrograph:** Energy is gained by a molecule as it is hit by photons. Some energy is re-emitted at different wavelengths. This decrease in wavelength is the property of the individual molecule
  - Rapid. (Can create capnograph)
- **Photoacoustic spectrometry:** Uses ultrasound and can create capnograph
- **Gas chromatography:** Can't do continuous measurements of CO_2, just single readings only

Renal replacement therapy

- Indications for renal replacement therapy (RRT) are
  - *Acute kidney injury (AKI) with*
    - Fluid overload (refractory to diuretics)

- ◆ Hyperkalaemia (K+ >6.5)
- ◆ Severe metabolic acidosis (pH <7.1)
- ◆ **Symptomatic uraemia:** Encephalopathy, pericarditis, bleeding, nausea
- ◆ Oliguria/anuria
- ◆ Toxins

- **Convection:** Movement of solute along with solvent resulting from bulk movement of fluid
- **Dialysis:** Diffusion of solute across a semi-permeable membrane down their concentration gradients
- **Drugs that are removed or not removed by RRT**

Removed	Not removed
Ethylene glycol	Digoxin
Methanol	Beta-blockers
Lithium	Tricyclic antidepressants
Salicylates	Phenytoin
Barbiturates	Benzodiazepines
Metformin	Gliclazide

- **Types of RRT in use in intensive care**
  - ○ **Intermittent haemodialysis (IHD):** Dialysis with high flow rates. Only in hemodynamically stable patients
  - ○ **Continuous renal replacement therapies (CRRTs)**
    - a. **Continuous venovenous haemodialysis (CVVHD):** Mode for removal of solutes of small molecular weight (e.g., urea, creatinine, potassium)
    - b. **Continuous venovenous haemofiltration (CVVH):** Mode for removal of small molecular weight solutes plus fluid removal
    - c. **Continuous venovenous haemodiafiltration (CVVHDF):** Clearance of solute of both small and medium molecular weight substances along with fluid
    - d. **Slow continuous ultrafiltration (SCUF):** Effective for safe management of fluid removal but doesn't allow significant solute clearance
  - ○ **Hybrid therapies:** For example, sustained low-efficiency dialysis (SLED). Daily but longer sessions. Solute and fluid removal are faster than CVVH but with hemodynamic stability like CVVH

Molecule to be removed	Size of molecule (Da)	Example	Preferred mode
Small molecules/ Electrolytes	<500	Urea, creatinine	Dialysis or filtration
Middle molecules	500–5000	Drugs	Filtration better than dialysis
Low molecular weight proteins	5000–50,000	Cytokines, complement	Filtration
Water	18		Filtration better than dialysis

Ultrasound

- **Principle:** Ultrasound waves are sound waves above the threshold of human hearing (2 MHz). They are produced by applying an electrical field to piezoelectric crystals (commonly ceramic lead zirconate titanate). These crystals in transducers vibrate and emit ultrasound waves. These waves are transmitted and reflected back to the transducer depending upon the density of tissue. These crystals change these waves back to electrical energy which are displayed on a monitor
  - **Highly reflective tissues/hyperechoic:** Bone (white)
  - **Weakly reflective tissues/hypoechoic:** Muscles and fat (grey)
  - **No reflection/anechoic:** Blood (black)
- **Speed of ultrasound in tissues:** 1540 m/s
  - **Speed in air:** 330 m/s
  - **Speed in bone:** 4080 m/s
- **Ultrasound frequencies used in medical scanners:** 2–20 MHz. Image is optimised by changing frequency. **Longer wavelengths penetrate greater depth**
  - **Gain function:** Digitally enhances the image. Signal amplification
- **Modes of ultrasound**
  - **A (amplitude)-mode:** Basic form. Measures the amplitude of reflected ultrasound waves reflected at each depth from the ultrasound probes. These amplitudes are displayed in the form of spike on a cathode ray oscilloscope (CRO), e.g., for ophthalmologists to measure diameter of the eyeball

○ **B (brightness)-mode/Two-dimensional (2D) mode:** In the brightness mode, signals from returning echoes are displayed as dots of varying intensities. The spike of the A-mode is replaced by a small dot on the CRO. The intensity of brightness of a dot is a relative measure of reflected light size. Different dot lines are produced for different distances from the transducer producing a 2D image

○ **M (Motion)-mode:** It uses rapid B-mode imaging to measure movement of anatomical structures, e.g., echocardiography

○ **Doppler mode:** Doppler imaging uses the Doppler effect of **change in frequency** caused by the motion of an object relative to a receiver. Sound waves are reflected from a moving object (blood). Thus, we can measure the wavelength of sound waves that are returned. **This gives us the direction as well as velocity of blood.** Red means direction towards the probe (like a bull towards a red cloth), blue means direction away from the probe

• **Doppler equation**

○ Velocity of moving target = $\dfrac{c \times \Delta f}{2f}$

where c = speed of sound wave

Δf = Change in frequency

f = Frequency

○ Doppler affects all kinds of waves

Magnetic resonance imaging

• **Magnetic resonance imaging (MRI):** Scanner used to visualize soft tissue.

• **Principle:** Protons present in hydrogen ions of water **(odd number of nucleons)** and fat molecules align in the direction of the magnetic field whenever a patient enters the MRI scanner

○ This magnetic field is produced by the passing of current through the coils of wire known as the **primary magnet**

○ **These coils of wires are cooled by liquid helium**

○ A second magnetic field is generated at right angles to these aligned protons

○ This disrupts the alignment of aligned protons and gives them a different axis known as nuclear precession

○ When the second electromagnetic field is removed, the protons return to their original level emitting some radiofrequency radiation in the process

○ This radiofrequency radiation, which is very small, is converted into an image

- o **Gradient magnet:** Small magnets that help to fine-tune the image of the area being studied. The sound of these magnets being turned on and off causes a banging noise in the MRI
- o 'T' is relaxation time constant. T1 is the image generated a few milliseconds after the electromagnetic field and T2 is image generated slightly later
- o **Faraday cage:** Room in which scanner is planted. Made of copper or aluminium
- Facts: Noise level >85 dB
  - o Earth's magnetic field = 1 Gauss
  - o 1 Tesla = 10,000 Gauss
  - o Commercial MRIs have the strength of 3T
  - o Tesla is the SI unit for magnetic flux density or Weber/m^2
  - o Weber is the SI unit for magnetic flux
  - o **50 Gauss line:** All ferromagnetic items will be subject to movement inside this line
- MRI equipment
  - o **MR safe:** Items that pose no hazard in any MR environment
  - o **MR conditional:** Items that are safe under certain tested magnetic conditions
  - o **MR unsafe:** Items that pose a hazard in any MR environment
- Problems with MRI
  - o Remote area anaesthesia problems
  - o Monitoring issues due to special equipment needed
  - o Claustrophobic environment to the patient
  - o Noisy environment
  - o Limited access to the patient and anaesthetic equipment
  - o Injury due to ferrous implants
  - o Injury due to burns produced by magnetically induced currents
  - o **Pacemakers are contraindicated**

LASER

- LASER: Light amplification by stimulated emission of radiation
  - o **Monochromatic, coherent and non-divergent**
  - o Wavelength dependent upon medium used
- Mechanism of generation
  - o Lasing medium (gas, liquid, solid, semiconductor)

- o High-voltage light stimulates the medium to generate a photon
- o Photon causes an electron in the excitable state to fall to the stable state releasing another photon in parallel and in phase
- o Mirror reflects photons back into lasing medium and amplification occurs
- Different types of lasing mediums
  - o Argon
    - ◆ Blue-green 400–700 nm
    - ◆ **Photocoagulation:** Ophthalmology, dermatology
    - ◆ 2-mm penetration
  - o **Carbon dioxide**
    - ◆ Infrared (10,600 nm) leads to vaporisation of water
    - ◆ Precision cutting with haemostasis, low penetration 0.2 mm (ENT, Neuro)
    - ◆ Cannot be used endoscopically
  - o **Neodymium doped yttrium aluminium garnet (Nd:YAG)**
    - ◆ Near-infrared 1064 nm
    - ◆ Not absorbed by water
    - ◆ Coagulation and deep penetration cutting 2–10 mm (tumor debulking)
  - o **Excimer ultraviolet (UV) laser**
    - ◆ Breaks chemical bonds, doesn't heat
    - ◆ Refractive surgery
- LASER classification in terms of safety
  - o Safe under all conditions of normal use
  - o Safe because blink reflex limits exposure, e.g., laser pointers
  - o Hazardous to the eye
  - o Can burn skin and cause devastating visual loss even when reflected (output >500 mW)
  - o Not safe when using visual aids, e.g., loupes

Fibreoptic scopes

- A **fibreoptic scope** is a flexible optical fibre bundle with an eyepiece on one end and a lens on the other and is used to inspect difficult-to-reach places such as the insides of the human body. It uses the principle of total internal reflection

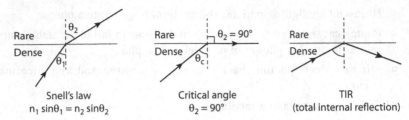

Figure 15.4 Critical angle.

- **Total internal reflection:** Optical phenomenon in which waves arriving at the interface from one medium to another are not refracted into the second medium, but are completely reflected back into the first medium
- For total internal reflection to happen, certain conditions must be met
  - The light is in the denser medium and approaching the less dense medium
  - The angle of incidence of the light ray must exceed the critical angle of the interface
- **Critical angle:** The angle of incidence that yields an angle of refraction of 90 degrees
- **Components of fibreoptic scopes**
  - **Eyepiece lens:** At the proximal end for viewing image
  - **Imaging bundle:** Continuous strand of flexible glass fibres that transmit the image to the eyepiece
  - **Distal lens:** The combination of micro lenses that take images and focus them into the small imaging bundle
  - **Illumination system:** Light system that relays light from the source to the target area
  - Channels for suction, instruments

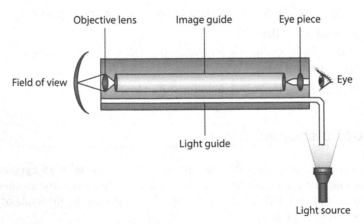

Figure 15.5 Fibreoptic scopes.

Statistics

16

Data and its distribution

Types of data

- Categorical (qualitative) data
  - Nominal: No numerically significant order, e.g., hair colour, blood groups
  - Ordinal: Order of magnitude, e.g., pain scores, American Society of Anaesthesiologists (ASA) score
- Numerical (quantitative) data
  - Discrete: Finite values, e.g., number of children
  - Continuous: Data that can take any number, e.g., height, age
  - Ratio: Data series that has zero as its baseline value, e.g., Kelvin temperature scale, blood pressure
  - Interval: Data series that includes zero on a larger scale e.g., Centigrade temperature scale

Measures of central tendency

- Mean: The average value
- Median: Middle value of a data series
- Mode: Frequently occurring value in a set of data points

Measures of spread

- Variance: A measure of the spread of data around a central point
$$Var = \sum (x - \bar{x})2/n$$
- Standard deviation: *A measure of the spread of data around a central point. **Square root of variance***
$$SD = \sqrt{\sum(xi - \bar{x})2/n\text{-}1}$$
- Standard error of the mean: A measure of the spread of a group of sample means around the true population mean
$$SEM = \sigma/\sqrt{N}\text{-}1$$

DOI: 10.1201/9781003390244-19

- **Confidence Intervals (CIs):** Range of values that will contain the true population mean with a stated percentage confidence. **95.4% CI is ±2 standard deviation (SD)**
  - 68.3% of values within 1 SD of the mean
  - 99.7% of values within 3 SD of the mean
- **Interquartile range:** The range of values that lie between the first and third quartiles, therefore, showing 50% of the data points. Best option for non-parametric data

Types of distribution

- **Normal distribution:** A bell-shaped distribution in which mean, median and mode all have the same value
- **Positively skewed distribution:** Longer tail stretching off towards the more positive values
  - Mean > median > mode
- **Negatively skewed distribution:** Longer tail stretching off towards the more negative values
  - Mode > median > mean

Type 1 and type 2 errors

- ***p* stands for probability:** Therefore, if $p = 1$, the event will always happen and if $p = 0$ the event will never happen
- **Null hypothesis:** Assumption is made that there is no significant difference between the means of the samples. If the result of the test gives a p <0.05, then there is a low possibility (5%) that the difference has occurred purely by chance and the null hypothesis that there is no difference between the sample is rejected
- **Type 1 error/α error:** It occurs when a null hypothesis is wrongly rejected
  - Lower the p value and the larger the sample size the smaller the chance of making a type 1 error
  - 5% chance of making a type 1 error is accepted
- **Type 2 error/β error:** It occurs when a null hypothesis is wrongly accepted
  - 20% chance of making a type 2 error is accepted
  - Three factors that increase the chance of making type 2 error
    - Large variability in study population
    - Small population size
    - Situation where a small difference is clinically important

- Power of a study: Likelihood of detecting a difference between groups if that difference really does exist
  - Power is probability of avoiding a type 2 error
  - Power = $1 - \beta$

Significance tests

- There are four considerations that should be taken into account
  - Data is qualitative or quantitative
  - Data is parametric or non-parametric
  - Two groups or more than two groups
  - Data paired or unpaired

	Two groups		More than two groups	
Type of data	Unpaired	Paired	Unpaired	Paired
Parametric (Continuous)	Student's unpaired t-test	Student's paired t-test	ANOVA	Paired ANOVA
Non-parametric (Nominal)	Chi-square test	McNemar's test	Chi-square test	Chi-square test
Non-parametric (Ordinal)	Mann–Whitney *U* test	Wilcoxon signed rank test	Kruskal–Wallis test	Friedman test

- Fisher's exact test: It is a variation of the chi-square test that is used when the value of parameters in any cell is less than 5
- Correlation: Degree of association between two variables
  - **Pearson's correlation coefficient:** Used for normally distributed data
  - **Spearman's rank correlation coefficient:** Used for non-normally distributed continuous data, for ordinal data or for data with relevant outliers
- Positive correlation: r value between 0 and +1
- Negative correlation: r value between 0 and –1
- No correlation: r value is 0

Change in peak expiratory flow or blood pressure can be a good example of student's paired t-test.

Sensitivity and specificity

	Diseased	Healthy
Positive	True positive (TP)	False positive (FP)
Negative	False negative (FN)	True negative (TN)

- **Sensitivity:** Probability that someone who has the disease tests positive
  - Numbers correctly positive/total number that is actually positive
  - True positive (TP)/TP + false negative (FN)
  - A test with high sensitivity is said to have a low type II error rate
- **Specificity:** Probability that someone who doesn't have the disease tests negative
  - Number correctly negative/total number that is actually negative
  - True negative (TN)/TN + false positive (FP)
  - A test with high specificity is said to have a low type I error rate
    - Both sensitivity and specificity are prevalence independent
- **Positive predictive value (PPV):** The certainty with which a positive test results correctly predicts a positive value
  - Numbers correctly positive/total number that tested positive
  - TP/TP + FP
- **Negative predictive value (NPV):** The certainty with which a negative test results correctly predicts a negative value
  - Numbers correctly negative/total number that tested negative
  - TN/TN + FN
    - Both PPV and NPV are influenced by prevalence of the disease

Odds ratio and number needed to treat

	Non-event (people relieved of pain)	Event (people in pain)
Painkiller	b	a
Placebo	d	c

- Painkiller events odd = event/non-event = a/b

Placebo events odd = event/non-event = c/d

- **Odds ratio** = painkiller events odd/placebo events odd = a ÷ b/c ÷ d
  - Odds of having the outcome
- **Relative risk** = risk of event in painkiller group/risk of event in placebo = a ÷ a + b/c ÷ c + d
  - Risk of developing the outcome
- Odds/risk ratio above 1 = your exposure increases risk of event occurring
- Odds/risk ratio below 1 = your exposure increases risk of event occurring or protective effect of exposure
- If 95% CI includes value 1, then there is no statistical difference
  - Wide CI = weaker inference
  - Narrow CI = stronger inference
- **Absolute risk reduction (ARR)** = event rate in placebo group – event rate in treatment group = c/c + d – a/a + b
- **Numbers needed to treat (NNT):** Number of patients that would need to be treated to prevent a single event. NNT = 1/ARR

Clinical trial

- Preclinical studies
  - In vitro studies
  - Animal studies

Phase	Number of people involved	Main aims of trial	Randomisation
0	10–20 people	• Single subtherapeutic doses • Preliminary data on pharmacokinetics and pharmacodynamics • No data on safety and efficacy	No
1	20–50 people	• Finding the best dose of treatment • Assesses safety of drug	No

(*Continued*)

Phase	Number of people involved	Main aims of trial	Randomisation
		• Tolerability • Pharmacokinetics • Pharmacodynamics	
2	Over 100	• Checking the best dose of treatment • More about safety of drug • Some phase 2 trials are randomised	Sometimes
3	Around thousands	• Comparing the new treatment to the standard treatment or to a dummy drug • At least 2 randomised controlled trials for approval	Usually
4	Market	• Post-marketing surveillance • Long-term benefits and side effects	No

Double blinding is to both investigator and participant.

Evidence-based medicine

Evidence-based medicine: Conscientious, explicit and judicious use of current evidence in making decisions about the care of individual patients

Level	Evidence
1a	Systemic review or meta-analysis of more than one randomised controlled trial (multiple RCTs)
1b	Single RCT
2a	Non-randomised study
2b	Cohort study/quasi-experimental study
3	Case-control study/
4	Case series
5	Expert opinion

Grade of recommendations

Grade	Recommendation
A	Consistent level 1 studies
B	Consistent level 2 or level 3 studies or extrapolations from level 1 studies
C	Level 4 studies or extrapolations from level 2 or level 3 studies
D	Level 5 evidence

- **Systematic review:** It answers a defined research question by collecting and summarising all empirical evidence that fits pre-specified eligibility criteria
  - Meta-analysis may or may not be used to analyse the results of the studies
- **Meta-analysis:** Uses statistical methods to summarize the results of these studies. Represented by a forest plot

ANATOMY

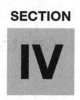

Anatomy

17

Brachial plexus

- **Brachial plexus:** Nerve plexus to the upper limb
  - **Roots:** Anterior rami of spinal nerves C5-T1
    - Lies in interscalene groove
  - **Trunks:** C5 and C6 combine to form superior trunk, C7 forms the middle trunk and C8 and T1 together form the inferior trunk
    - Between anterior and middle scalene muscles
  - **Divisions:** Each division splits into an anterior and posterior division
    - Passes behind the clavicle
  - **Cords:** The lateral cord is formed by combination of anterior divisions of the superior and middle trunk. The medial cord is formed by continuation of anterior division of the inferior trunk. The posterior cord is formed by coming together of posterior divisions of superior, middle and inferior trunks
    - Cords lie in axilla
  - **Terminal branches:** Musculocutaneous, axillary, radial, median and ulnar nerves are terminal branches
- Nerves with muscles supplied
  - **Long thoracic:** C5–C7, serratus anterior
  - **Thoracodorsal:** C6–C8, latissimus dorsi
  - **Dorsal scapular:** C5, levator scapulae and rhomboids

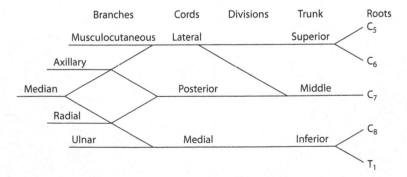

Figure 17.1 Brachial plexus.

DOI: 10.1201/9781003390244-21

○ **Suprascapular:** C5–C6, supraspinatus and infraspinatus

○ **Lateral pectoral:** C5–C7, pectoralis major and minor

○ **Medial pectoral:** C8–T1, pectoralis major and minor

○ **Upper subscapular:** C5–C6, subscapularis

○ **Lower subscapular:** C5–C6, subscapularis and Teres major

Lumbar plexus

- **Lumbar plexus:** Nerve plexus to the upper limb formed by anterior rami of spinal nerve roots L1–L4 along with variable contribution of T12
  ○ Plexus is formed within the psoas muscle
  ○ The nerves of the lumbar plexus pass in front of the hip joint and mainly support the anterior part of the thigh
- **Iliohypogastric:** *T12, L1* – Emerges from the upper lateral border of the psoas major muscle and in front of the quadratus lumborum muscle. Pierces transversus abdominis muscle to lie within the transversus abdominis plane
  ○ Sensory innervation to the skin of the posterolateral gluteal and suprapubic regions
  ○ Motor supply to transversus abdominis, internal abdominal oblique, conjoint tendon
- **Ilioinguinal:** *T12, L1* – Emerges from the upper lateral border of the psoas major muscle and in front of the quadratus lumborum muscle, just below the iliohypogastric nerve. Pierces transversus abdominis muscle to lie within the transversus abdominis plane
  ○ Sensory innervation to the skin of the upper anteromedial thigh and partially the external genitalia
  ○ Motor supply to transversus abdominis and internal abdominal oblique muscles
- **Genitofemoral:** *L1, L2* – The nerve originates in the substance of the psoas major muscle and descends retroperitoneally towards the inguinal ligament
  ○ Genital branch enters the inguinal canal via the deep ring. Motor supply to cremasteric muscle. Sensory supply to anterior scrotal area/ mons pubis and labia majora
  ○ Femoral branch provides sensation to the skin overlying the femoral triangle
- **Femoral nerve:** *L2,3,4* – Largest terminal branch. Lies between psoas and iliacus muscles Travels below the inguinal ligament
  ○ Sensory innervation to anterior thigh and medial lower leg and **saphenous nerve**
  ○ Motor supply to quadriceps femoris (extensors of the knee) and pectineus, sartorius, iliacus **(flexors of hip)**

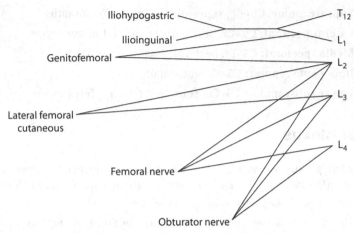

Figure 17.2 Lumbar plexus.

- **Obturator nerve: *L2,3,4*** – Originates from medial border of psoas. Enters the thigh through the obturator foramen
    - Sensory supply to skin of medial thigh and articular branch for the hip and knee joints
    - Motor innervation to all the medial muscles of the thigh (hip adductors) except for the hamstring part of the adductor magnus
- **Lateral cutaneous nerve of thigh: *L2,3*** – Emerges lateral to Iliacus muscle. Passes below the inguinal ligament. Sensory supply to skin of the lateral thigh

Movement	Myotome
Shoulder abduction	C5
Elbow flexion, wrist extension	C6
Elbow extension	C7
Thumb extension and wrist ulnar deviation	C8
Finger abduction	T1
Hip flexion	L2
Knee extension	L3
Ankle dorsiflexion	L4
Big toe extension	L5
Ankle plantarflexion	S1
Knee flexion	S2

Sacral plexus

- **Sacral plexus:** Derived from the anterior rami of spinal nerves L4–L5 and S1–S4
  - Located on the posterior pelvic wall, posterior to the internal iliac vessels and ureter and anterior to the piriformis muscle
  - All branches leave the pelvis via the greater sciatic foramen
- **Superior gluteal nerve:** *L4–5, S1* – Supplies the motor function of the gluteus medius, gluteus minimus and tensor fasciae latae
- **Inferior gluteal nerve:** *L5, S1–2:* – Supplies motor function to gluteus maximus
- **Posterior cutaneous nerve of the thigh:** Supplies sensation to gluteal region, perineum and posterior thigh and leg
- **Sciatic nerve:** Largest nerve in the human body. Descends between greater trochanter of femur and ischial tuberosity
  - It descends through the posterior compartment of the thigh
  - Before entering the popliteal fossa, the nerve into two large terminal branches, the tibial nerve and common fibular (peroneal) nerve
- **Tibial nerve:** It passes deep to the fibular and tibial heads of the soleus muscle into the deep layer of the posterior compartment of the leg, along with the posterior tibial vessels
  - The tibial nerve exits the posterior compartment of the leg at the ankle joint, passing behind the medial malleolus to enter the sole of the foot and divides into medial and lateral plantar nerves
  - **Motor supply: (plantar flexion)**
    - Superficial leg muscles like gastrocnemius, soleus, plantaris and popliteus
    - Deep leg muscle group like tibialis posterior, flexor hallucis longus and flexor digitorum longus
    - The articular branches provide innervation to the knee joint, superior and inferior tibiofibular joints and the ankle joint
    - **Medial plantar nerve:** Abductor hallucis, flexor digitorum brevis, flexor hallucis brevis, first lumbrical
    - **Lateral plantar nerve:** Quadratus plantae, flexor digiti minimi, adductor hallucis, the interossei, three lumbricals and abductor digiti minimi
  - **Sensory supply:** Injury causes tarsal tunnel syndrome
    - Sural nerve supplies the skin of the posterolateral leg and lateral foot

- Medial plantar nerve is to the anterior two-thirds of the medial sole and medial three and one-half toes, including the nail beds on the dorsum
- Lateral plantar nerve supplies the anterior two-thirds of the lateral sole and lateral one and one-half toes
- **Common fibula nerve:** Enters the anterior compartment of the leg by winding around the head of the fibula
  - The nerve divides into the superficial fibular nerve and deep fibular nerve
  - **Motor supply:** Injury causes foot drop
    - The superficial fibular nerve supplies the muscles of the lateral compartment of the leg like fibularis longus and fibularis brevis
    - **The deep fibular nerve** supplies the muscles of the anterior compartment of the leg like tibialis anterior, extensor hallucis longus, extensor digitorum longus and the dorsum of the foot like extensor digitorum brevis, extensor hallucis brevis. **(Dorsiflexion of foot)**
    - The articular branches that innervate the ankle joint, tarsal and metatarsophalangeal joints
  - **Sensory supply:** The superficial fibular nerve provides sensation to the anterolateral aspect of the leg and dorsal aspects of foot and toes
    - The deep fibular branch innervates a portion of the skin between the first and second toes
    - A small sensory branch, the lateral sural cutaneous nerve provides sensation inferolaterally to the knee

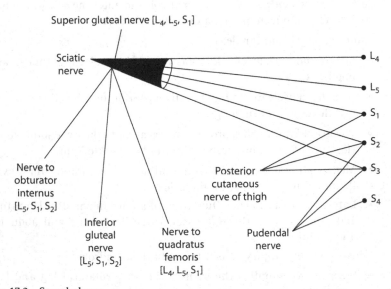

Figure 17.3 Sacral plexus.

Upper limb nerve blocks

Approach	Sensory block	Complications	Remarks
Interscalene (Roots)	Shoulder, upper arm, elbow	- **Phrenic nerve palsy (90%), Horner's syndrome (20%),** recurrent laryngeal nerve block (15%), subarachnoid injection, vertebral artery puncture	- Ulnar nerve may be spared - Suprascapular nerve may be missed - USG sign: *Traffic light sign* - Anatomic landmark: Palpate for interscalene groove at level of cricoid cartilage C6
Supraclavicular (Trunks and divisions)	Entire arm	- Pneumothorax, phrenic nerve palsy (40–60%), Horner's syndrome (70–90%)	- Ulnar nerve may be spared - Suprascapular nerve may be missed - USG sign: *Bunch of grapes* - Anatomic landmark: 1 cm above midclavicular point lateral to subclavian artery pulsation
Infraclavicular (Cords)	Forearm, wrist, hand	- Pneumothorax, Intravascular injection	- Landmarks may be difficult
Axillary (Terminal branches)	Forearm, wrist, hand	- Haematoma formation, intravascular injection - **Retained sensation over lateral forearm due to musculocutaneous being missed**	- **Musculocutaneous nerve** may be spared - Intercostobrachial nerve may be missed
Median	Radial side of palm	- Median nerve damage: Thenar muscle wasting and numbness of hand or **hand of benediction**	- Blocked at wrist: Between flexor carpi radialis and palmaris longus
Musculocuta-neous	Lateral cutaneous nerve of the forearm	- Musculocutaneous damage: Weakness of arm flexion and sensory loss along the lateral forearm	- At level of cubital fossa: Subcutaneous local anaesthetic between biceps and brachioradialis

(*Continued*)

Approach	Sensory block	Complications	Remarks
Radial	Lateral, radial side of the hand and forearm	- Radial nerve damage - At level of axilla: **Crutch palsy** or **Saturday night palsy** - At level of mid humerus: **Wrist drop**	- Blocked at wrist - Field block over wrist over anatomical snuff box
Ulnar	Medial side of the hand and forearm	- Ulnar nerve damage: **Claw hand** - *Positive Froment's sign*	Blocked at the wrist: Just above styloid process and under tendon of flexor carpi ulnaris

At antecubital fossa: Median nerve can get damaged while doing intravenous cannulation.

Lower limb nerve blocks

Approach	Sensory block	Remarks	Landmarks
Sciatic nerve	- Surgery at and below level of knee	- Sciatic nerve block may be a useful adjunct for certain lower extremity chronic pain syndromes such as sciatic neuropathy or piriformis syndrome where there is compression of the sciatic nerve at the piriformis muscle	- **Classic approach of Labat:** A line is drawn from the greater trochanter to the posterior superior iliac spine. From the midpoint of this line, a perpendicular is dropped 3–5 cm - **Anterior approach** - **Posterior approach** - **Lateral approach** - **Popliteal fossa approach:** A line is drawn vertically for about 7 cm from the midpoint of the skin crease and injection is made about 1 cm lateral to this point

(Continued)

Approach	Sensory block	Remarks	Landmarks
Lumbar plexus	- Hip or femoral operations including knee	- Anterior approach for lumbar plexus is sometimes called a 3-in-1	- **Posterior approach:** Draw two lines, one parallel to the spinous processes passing through the posterior superior iliac spine, and the other joining the highest points of both iliac crests (L3–L4). The point of needle insertion is at the intersection of these two lines
Femoral nerve	- Surgery on femur, anterior thigh and knee	- Combined with a sciatic nerve block to provide lower extremity coverage below the knee	- The needle is inserted approximately 1 cm lateral to the femoral artery pulse in a cephalad direction
3-in-1 block (femoral, obturator, lateral femoral cutaneous nerve block)	- Cannulated hip screws	- Doesn't provide reliable analgesia above level of the greater trochanter	- 1 cm lateral to femoral pulse and 2 cm below inguinal ligament - Large volume of local anaesthetic is used
Fascia iliaca block (femoral, obturator, lateral femoral cutaneous nerve block)	- Analgesia to fracture neck of femur in emergency department	- Alternative to standard 3-in-1 block	- 1 cm inferior to line joining pubic tubercle and anterior superior iliac spine (ASIS) - Two pops are heard as it passes through fascia lata and then fascia iliaca

(*Continued*)

Approach	Sensory block	Remarks	Landmarks
Lateral femoral cutaneous nerve block	- Skin grafts and surgery of outer thigh	- Meralgia paraesthetica: Entrapment of the lateral cutaneous nerve of the thigh is caused by compression of the nerve near the ASIS and the inguinal ligament	- Beneath fascia lata, 2 cm medial and inferior to ASIS
Adductor canal (saphenous nerve)	- Knee arthro-plasty	- It doesn't cause motor block of femoral nerve - Early ambulation	- Adductor canal formed by sartorius (superiorly), vastus medialis (laterally), adductor longus and magnus (medially)
Ankle block	- Anaes-thesia and postopera-tive analgesia for awake forefoot surgery	- Block the tibial nerve first, as this nerve block takes the longest time to develop - Useful for daycare surgeries	- **Posterior tibial:** Behind middle malleolus - **Sural:** Behind lateral malleolus - **Superficial peroneal:** Above lateral malleolus - **Deep peroneal:** Between extensor hallucis longus and dorsalis pedis - **Saphenous:** 5 cm above medial malleolus

Truncal nerve blocks

Block	Position	Plane of injection	Indications	Complications
TAP block (lateral approach)	Midpoint between subcostal margin and iliac crest in mid-axillary line	Internal oblique and transversus abdominis	Lower abdominal/pelvic surgeries, e.g., lower segment Caesarean section (LSCS)	Intraperitoneal injection and intestinal puncture

(Continued)

Block	Position	Plane of injection	Indications	Complications
TAP block (subcostal approach)	Subcostal in midclavicular line	Rectus abdominis and transversus abdominis	Upper abdominal surgeries with subcostal margin	Intraperitoneal injection and liver trauma
Rectus sheath block	Subcostal in paramedian	Rectus abdominis and posterior rectus sheath	Abdominal surgeries with midline incision	Wound infection and catheter migration to intraperitoneal space
Quadratus lumborum	Above iliac crest in the back, para median	Quadratus lumborum and psoas major	Lower abdominal surgeries such as nephrectomy	Catheter migration to retroperitoneal space
Serratus anterior block	Mid-axillary line, at the level of the nipple	Latissimus dorsi and serratus anterior	Anterolateral, or lateral rib fractures	Vascular puncture and pleural puncture
Erector spinae plane block	T5–T7 paraspinal fascial plane	Erector spinae muscle and the thoracic transverse processes	Posterior rib fractures and thoracotomies	Vascular puncture and pleural puncture
Ilioinguinal Iliohypogas-tric	Near anterior superior iliac spine	Internal oblique and transversus abdominis	Inguinal hernia repair	Intraperitoneal injection and femoral nerve block
Genitofemoral (spermatic cord block)	Along the inguinal ligament	Spermatic cord	Scrotal surgery	Vascular trauma
PECS block I	Mid-clavicular line, infraclavicular area	Pectoralis major and pectoralis minor	Breast surgery	Pneumothorax and trauma to vessels

(*Continued*)

Block	Position	Plane of injection	Indications	Complications
PECS block II	Anterior axillary line, over third rib	Pectoralis minor and serratus anterior	Breast surgery with axillary dissection	Pneumothorax and trauma to vessels
Paravertebral block	Lateral to spinous processes	Superior costotransverse ligament and pleura	Breast, thoracic wall and chest wall surgeries	Pneumothorax and epidural spread of the local anaesthetic (LA)
Intercostal nerve block	6–7 cm lateral to spinous process	Internal intercostal and the innermost intercostal muscles	Analgesia for upper thoracic surgeries and chest trauma	Pneumothorax

Diaphragm

- Dome-shaped fibromuscular structure, central tendinous and peripheral muscular
- **Attachments**
  - ○ **Vertebral part:** Right and left crura attaches to anterior vertebral bodies (L1–L3)
    - ♦ Median ligament attaches the two crura
  - ○ **Medial arcuate ligament:** Thickening of psoas fascia
  - ○ **Lateral arcuate ligament:** Thickening of quadratus lumborum fascia
  - ○ **Coastal part:** Six lowest ribs and costal cartilage
  - ○ **Sternal part:** Xiphisternum
- **Foramina**
  - ○ **T8:** Inferior vena cava (IVC) and right phrenic nerve
  - ○ **T10:** Oesophagus and vagus nerves
  - ○ **T12:** Aorta, azygos vein, thoracic duct
- **Nerve supply**
  - ○ **Motor:** Phrenic nerve (C3–C5)
  - ○ **Sensory:** Phrenic nerve and lower intercostals peripherally

- Blood supply
  - Superior phrenic artery: Thoracic aorta
  - Inferior phrenic artery: Abdominal aorta
  - Musculophrenic artery: Internal thoracic artery
  - Pericardiacophrenic artery: Internal thoracic artery
  - Lower internal intercostal arteries
- Hiatal hernia
  - **Sliding:** Oesophagus and stomach slide into thorax (reflux and dyspepsia)
  - **Rolling:** Fundus rolls into thorax but lower oesophagus remains intraabdominal (dyspepsia but no reflux)

Larynx

- Hyoid bone, *C-3; thyroid notch,* C-4; cricoid cartilage, C-6
- **Three paired cartilages:** Arytenoid, corniculate, cuneiform
- **Three unpaired cartilages:** Cricoid, thyroid, epiglottis
- Intrinsic muscles
  - **Cricothyroid:** Tenses vocal cords
  - **Vocalis:** Alters vocal folds
  - **Posterior cricoarytenoid:** Abducts vocal cords
  - **Lateral cricoarytenoid:** Adducts vocal cords
  - **Transverse arytenoid:** Closes rima glottidis
  - **Oblique arytenoid:** Closes rima glottidis
  - **Thyroarytenoid:** Relaxes vocal cords
- **Extrinsic muscle:**
  - Elevate larynx
    - Digastric
    - Mylohyoid
    - Stylohyoid
    - Geniohyoid
  - Depresses larynx
    - Sternohyoid
    - Thyrohyoid
    - Sternothyroid
    - Omohyoid

- Nerve supply
  - Superior laryngeal nerve → internal laryngeal nerve → sensory innervation above level of vocal cords
  - Superior laryngeal nerve → external laryngeal nerve → innervates cricothyroid muscle
  - Recurrent laryngeal nerve → sensory innervation below the level of vocal cords + all intrinsic muscles of larynx except cricothyroid
- Blood supply
  - Superior laryngeal artery branch of superior thyroid artery
  - Inferior laryngeal artery branch of inferior thyroid artery
  - Superior and inferior laryngeal veins
- **Recurrent laryngeal nerve:** Right-sided loops under subclavian artery, left-sided loops under arch of aorta
  - **Unilateral palsy:** Hoarseness of voice
  - **Bilateral palsy:**
    - **Complete:** Neutral position
    - **Partial:** Stridor as abductors are more affected by weakness (Semon's law)
- **Superior laryngeal nerve damage:** Hoarseness, risk of aspiration

Base of skull

Foramina	Structures passing through it
Cribriform plate	- Olfactory nerve (cranial nerve [CN] I)
Greater palatine foramen	- Greater palatine nerve - Descending palatine vessels
Optic canal	- Optic nerve (CN II) - Ophthalmic artery
Superior orbital fissure	- CNs III, IV and VI - Ophthalmic branch of trigeminal nerve
Foramen rotundum	- Maxillary branch of trigeminal nerve
Foramen ovale	- Mandibular branch of trigeminal nerve
Foramen spinosum	- Nervus spinosus - Middle meningeal artery
Foramen lacerum/ Carotid canal	- Internal carotid artery

(Continued)

Foramina	Structures passing through it
Internal acoustic meatus	- Facial nerve (CN VII) - Vestibulocochlear nerve - Labyrinthine artery
Jugular foramen	- CNs IX, X, XI - Sigmoid sinus
Hypoglossal canal	- Hypoglossal nerve
Foramen magnum	- Spinal cord - Vertebral artery - Accessory nerve (CN XI)

Ganglion blockade

- **Stellate ganglion:** Sympathetic ganglion formed by fusion of inferior cervical and first thoracic ganglia
  - Sympathetic nerve supply to the head and neck as well as to the upper extremity is from stellate ganglion
  - Indications
    - **Neuropathic pain conditions:** Complex reginal pain syndrome (CRPS) I and II, post-herpetic neuralgia, phantom limb pain
    - **Ischaemic conditions:** Raynaud's disease, scleroderma, inadvertent intra-arterial injection in the upper limb
    - Refractory angina
    - Hyperhidrosis
    - Paget's disease of bone
  - **Techniques of blockade**
    - **Anterior approach:** Done at the C6 level (Chassaignac tubercle) after retracting the trachea and carotid pulse
    - **Paratracheal approach:** The needle is inserted two fingerbreadths lateral to the suprasternal notch and two fingerbreadths superior to the clavicle
  - **Complications:** Recurrent laryngeal nerve block, brachial plexus block, carotid or vertebral arterial puncture, intrathecal injection, pneumothorax. Block of stellate ganglion causes ipsilateral Horner's syndrome symptoms like ptosis, miosis, enophthalmos and anhidrosis
- **Coeliac plexus:** Largest sympathetic plexus. Lies near the root of the coeliac artery at the level of L1. Present bilaterally
  - Receives the greater splanchnic nerve (T5–T9), lesser splanchnic nerve (T9–T11) and the least splanchnic nerve (T11–T12) and supplies abdomen

- ○ Indications
  - ♦ *Malignant pain:* Pancreas cancer, stomach cancer
  - ♦ *Non-malignant pain:* Chronic pancreatitis
  - ♦ Diagnostic purposes
- ○ Techniques of blockade
  - ♦ *Posterior para-aortic:* Prone position. Using radiographical tools, the T12 and L1 vertebral bodies are identified. Approximately 6–8 cm from the midline, a spinal type needle is advanced at a 45-degree angle from posterior to anterior toward the ventral surface of the T12–L1 intervertebral space. Once the vertebral body has been contacted the spinal needle is advanced approximately another 1 cm further into the prevertebral fascial plane. Once the needle is in the desired position, confirm appropriate local by the spread of contrast under CT or fluoroscopic guidance
  - ♦ *Anterior para-aortic:* Supine position. With the patient in the supine position, the needle's trajectory is mapped via computed tomography (CT) or fluoroscopic guidance. Needle is inserted into the abdominal wall just anterior to the T12 vertebral body. The needle's course will typically encounter abdominal viscera including bowel, stomach or liver
- ○ Complications: Retroperitoneal bleeding, Intravascular injection into great vessels, paraplegia, visceral puncture, pneumothorax, chylothorax, diarrhoea, sexual dysfunction, orthostatic hypotension
- • **Lumbar sympathetic chain:** Lumbar sympathetic trunk lies on the fascial plane on the anterolateral aspect of the vertebral bodies
  - ○ Indications: Peripheral vascular disease, CRPS, phantom limb
  - ○ Technique: Posterior approach
    - ♦ *Prone:* The spinous process of L3 is identified with the image intensifier and a point marked 7–10 cm lateral to it. A needle is advanced under fluoroscopic guidance to the anterolateral edge of L3
  - ○ Complications: Puncture of aorta or IVC, inadvertent subarachnoid injection, genitofemoral neuritis, perforation of viscera

MISCELLANEOUS

SECTION

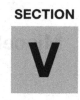

Miscellaneous

18

Numericals

- Calculate FiO$_2$ for a venturi mask
  - FiO$_2$ = $\dfrac{(\text{Airflow} \times 0.21) + (\text{Oxygen flow} \times 1.0)}{\text{Total flow}}$
  - So, for an entrainment ratio of 1:10 and O$_2$ flow rate of 6 L/min
  - Oxygen flow = 6 L, Airflow is 10 times = 60 L, Total flow = 66 L
  - $\dfrac{(60 \times 0.21) + (6 \times 1)}{66} = 0.28 = 28\%$

- A heated water bath contains 2 L of water at 25°C. Appliance shows 240 V, 0.4 A. The specific heat capacity of water is 4 kJ/kg/°C. **How long will it take for water to reach 35°C?**
  - Energy = mass × specific heat capacity × change in temperature
    - E = 2 × 4000 × 10 = 80,000 J
  - Power of appliance, P = IV, 0.4 × 240 = 96 W
  - Power = Energy/Time, 96 = 80,000/time, hence, time = 80,000/96 = 833.33 s

- **Weak acid with a pKa of 3.4. At a pH of 7.4, ratio of un-ionised to ionised drug**
  - pH = pKa + log $\dfrac{[\text{Conjugate base}]}{\text{Acid}}$
  - 7.4 = 3.4 + log $\dfrac{[\text{A}^-]}{\text{HA}}$ →→→ 4 = log $\dfrac{[\text{A}^-]}{\text{HA}}$ →→ Log 10^4 = Log $\dfrac{\text{Ionised}}{\text{Un-ionised}}$
  - Ionised/Un-ionised = 1/10^4

- **Plasma concentration of inulin is 35 µg/mL. Urine concentration is 3.5 mg/mL and total urine volume in 6 hours is 480 mL. What is the glomerular filtration rate (GFR)?**
  - Amount in urine = 3.5 × 480 = 1680 mg over 6 hours = 280 mg/hr = 4.6 mg/min = 4600 µg/min
  - GFR = $\dfrac{4600 \text{ µg/min}}{35 \text{ µg/mL}}$ = 131.42 mL/min

DOI: 10.1201/9781003390244-23

- pH of 0.05 M of sulphuric acid?
  - Ions of H^+ in 0.05 M sulphuric acid = 2×0.05 = 0.1 M
  - pH = $-Log_{10}[H^+]$ = $-Log_{10}0.1$ = 1
- A total of 200 subjects, 100 in a placebo group and 100 in drug group A. In the placebo group 10 subjects suffer a deep venous thrombosis (DVT). In the drug group A group 5 subjects suffer from DVT. What is the value of relative risk reduction?

	Event	No event
Drug A	5	95
Control	10	90

  - Odds ratio = $5/95 \div 10/90$ = 0.46
  - Relative risk = $5/100 \div 10/100$ = 0.5
  - Relative risk reduction = $5 - 10/10$ = $- 0.5$ = 50% reduction

Guidelines

- **Acute coronary syndrome (ACS):** Always give oxygen first
  - Aspirin and clopidogrel should be given as soon as possible if a diagnosis of ACS has been made
- **Post-dural puncture headache:** First thing is start by encouraging oral fluids intake
  - Caffeinated drinks
  - Simple analgesics
  - Epidural blood patch
- **Armitage formula:** For intraoperative and postoperative analgesia using caudal block
  - 0.25% bupivacaine ± adjuvant. Maximum dose of bupivacaine = 2 mg/kg
    - 0.5 mL/kg: Lumbosacral block
    - 1 mL/kg: Thoracolumbar block
    - 1.25 mL/kg: Midthoracic block
- **ALS guidelines for bradycardia:** *If hemodynamically unstable*, Mobitz type II block; *complete heart block*, recent asystole or ventricular pauses >3 s
  - Initial treatment is atropine, six doses of 0.5 mg intravenously (IV) each

- Adrenaline, isoprenaline infusion or transcutaneous pacing
- **Glucagon** in case of beta-blocker/calcium channel blocker poisoning
- Ultimately transvenous pacing needs to be done
- ALS guidelines for tachycardia
  - *If hemodynamically unstable*
    - Synchronised direct current (DC) shock, up to three attempts
    - Amiodarone 300 mg IV over 10–20 min, repeat synchronised DC shock
  - If hemodynamically stable
    - If QRS <0.12 s and regular, use vagal manoeuvres, adenosine 6 mg, 12 mg, 18 mg. If ineffective, give verapamil or beta-blocker
    - If QRS <0.12 s and irregular, control rate by beta-blocker or diltiazem. If heart failure considers digoxin or amiodarone. Anticoagulate if duration >48 hours
    - If QRS > 0.12 s and regular, If ventricular tachycardia (VT), use amiodarone 300 mg IV over 10–60 min. If previous supraventricular tachycardia (SVT) with bundle branch block (BBB), treat as regular narrow complex tachycardia
    - If QRS >0.12 s and irregular, If atrial fibrillation (AF) with BBB, treat as irregular narrow complex tachycardia. If polymorphic VT, give magnesium 2 g over 10 min
- Difficult airway guidelines: Adult patients
  - Plan A – *Tracheal intubation:* 3 + 1 (experienced colleague) intubation attempts
  - Plan B – *Oxygenation using supraglottic airway device (SAD) insertion:* Three attempts using a second-generation SAD
  - Plan C – *Face mask ventilation:* Use two-person technique
  - Plan D – *Emergency front of neck access:* Scalpel (#10 blade), bougie and tube (cuffed 6.0 mm ID) required
  - Capnography is gold standard for confirmation of endotracheal tube (ETT) placement
- World Health Organization (WHO) analgesic ladder
  - *Step 1:* Paracetamol + non-steroidal anti-inflammatory drugs (NSAIDs)
  - *Step 2:* Weak opioids like codeine phosphate, dihydrocodeine
  - *Step 3:* Strong opioids like morphine, fentanyl
  - *Step 4:* Nerve blocks, epidural, patient-controlled analgesia (PCA) pump

- Glasgow Coma Score
  - *Eye-opening response*
    - Spontaneously: 4
    - To speech: 3
    - To pain: 2
    - No response: 1
  - *Verbal response*
    - Oriented to time, person and place: 5
    - Confused: 4
    - Inappropriate words: 3
    - Incomprehensible sounds: 2
    - No response: 1
  - *Motor response*
    - Obeys command: 6
    - Moves to localize pain: 5
    - Flex to withdraw from pain: 4
    - Abnormal flexion: 3
    - Abnormal extension: 2
    - *No response:* 1

Index

Printed in the United States
by Baker & Taylor Publisher Services